Current Cancer Research

Series Editor
Wafik El-Deiry
Hershey, PA, USA

For further volumes:
http://www.springer.com/series/7892

Isabelle Mercier · Jean-François Jasmin
Michael P. Lisanti
Editors

Caveolins in Cancer Pathogenesis, Prevention and Therapy

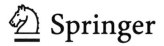

Editors
Isabelle Mercier
Department of Stem Cell Biology &
Regenerative Medicine
Thomas Jefferson University
Philadelphia, PA 19107, USA
isabelle.mercier@jefferson.edu

Jean-François Jasmin
Department of Stem Cell Biology &
Regenerative Medicine
Thomas Jefferson University
Philadelphia, PA 19107, USA
jeanfrancois.jasmin@jefferson.edu

Michael P. Lisanti
Department of Stem Cell Biology &
Regenerative Medicine
Thomas Jefferson University
Philadelphia, PA 19107, USA
mlisanti@KimmelCancerCenter.org

ISBN 978-1-4614-1000-3   e-ISBN 978-1-4614-1001-0
DOI 10.1007/978-1-4614-1001-0
Springer New York Dordrecht Heidelberg London

Library of Congress Control Number: 2011939408

Printed on acid-free paper

Springer is part of Springer Science+Business Media (www.springer.com)

Preface

Caveolae, a subset of lipid rafts, are flask-shaped invaginations of the plasma membrane that play an important role in cellular signal transduction by concentrating several molecules in a confined microenvironment. This clathrin-independent pathway of endocytosis is also involved in other crucial cellular processes, ranging from cholesterol transport to pathogen uptake. Caveolin (Cav) proteins, the main structural components of caveolae, are essential for maintaining caveolar integrity, as well as regulating cell signaling through protein–protein interactions. Cav proteins are composed of three distinct members, namely Cav-1, -2 and -3. However, Cav-1 still remains the best-studied and well-characterized member. More specifically, Cav-1 has been implicated in the pathogenesis of several human diseases such as atherosclerosis, heart disease, stroke, diabetes, and cancer, the latter being the focus of this book.

Most of the functional effects of Cav-1 are mediated through its scaffolding domain, which is located at amino acids 82–101. This domain recognizes a Cav binding motif found within signaling molecules, which can directly regulate their activities and downstream effects on cellular proliferation. Cav-1 primarily acts as a tumor suppressor in several types of human cancer and its downregulation correlates with cancer development and progression. In addition, mutations of the Cav-1 gene have been detected in tumor samples from cancer patients. One specific mutation of the Cav-1 gene results in the replacement of a proline for a leucine at amino acid position 132 (P132L). The Cav-1 (P132L) mutation can be detected in up to 16% of breast cancer specimens and acts as a dominant-negative mutant, which prevents the proper folding and expression of wild-type Cav-1. Recent studies have also reported a role for Cav-1 in tumor-associated stromal cells. Indeed, Cav-1 has been shown to directly regulate the behavior of cancer-associated fibroblasts (CAFs) isolated from invasive breast tumors.

Interestingly, the role of Cav-1 is not restricted to that of a tumor suppressor. Indeed, Cav-1 can also behave as a tumor promoter in certain types of tissues. For example, its over-expression has been associated with the development of aggressive tumors in some cancer patients. In these cases, Cav-1 can be secreted to mediate paracrine effects on neighboring epithelial cells, fibroblasts, and/or endothelial cells. In fact, a secreted form of Cav-1 has been detected in the serum of prostate cancer and melanoma patients and was recently proposed as a new predictive biomarker of tumor stage associated with poor clinical prognosis.

Due to the complex nature and tissue-specific functions of Cav proteins, there was a need for a reference book that summarized the literature and describes the future of these important proteins in the field of cancer research. As such, we brought together several experts in the field of Cavs and cancer to summarize the role of Cav-1 in six different epithelial cancers and the tumor-associated stroma, as well as its regulation of angiogenesis. We would like to thank all the authors who shared their scientific knowledge and opinions about the important roles of Cavs in cancer.

Philadelphia, PA, USA   Isabelle Mercier
Jean-François Jasmin
Michael P. Lisanti

Contents

1 Local and Distant Effects of Caveolin-1 on Prostate Cancer Progression 1
T.C. Thompson, S.A. Tahir, L. Li, M. Watanabe, K. Naruishi,
G. Yang, Ken-ichi Tabata, S. Kurosaka, K. Edamura,
R. Tanimoto, P. Corn, D. Kadmon, C.J. Logothetis,
P. Troncoso, C. Ren, A. Goltsov, and S. Park

2 Caveolin-1 in Colon Cancer: The Flexible Connection to Wnt Signaling 17
Andrew F.G. Quest, Vicente A. Torres, Diego A. Rodriguez,
Jorge Gutierrez-Pajares, and Julio C. Tapia

3 Caveolin-1 and Pancreatic Ductal Adenocarcinoma 43
David W. Rittenhouse, Oeendree Mukherjee, Nathan G. Richards,
Charles J. Yeo, Agnieszka K. Witkiewicz, and Jonathan R. Brody

4 Caveolin-1 in Brain Tumors 53
Rebecca Senetta and Paola Cassoni

5 The Role of Caveolin-1 in Skin Cancer 65
Alessandra Carè, Isabella Parolini, Federica Felicetti,
and Massimo Sargiacomo

6 Caveolins in Tumor Angiogenesis 75
Grzegorz Sowa

7 Caveolin-1 and Breast Cancer 91
Gloria Bonuccelli and Michael P. Lisanti

8 Caveolin-1 and Cancer-Associated Stromal Fibroblasts 105
Isabelle Mercier and Michael P. Lisanti

Index 121

Contributors

Gloria Bonuccelli Department of Stem Cell Biology & Regenerative Medicine, Thomas Jefferson University, Philadelphia, PA, USA

Jonathan R. Brody Department of Surgery, Jefferson Pancreas, Biliary and Related Cancer Center, and Kimmel Cancer Center, Thomas Jefferson University, Philadelphia, PA, USA

Department of Pathology, Thomas Jefferson University, Philadelphia, PA, USA

Alessandra Carè Department of Hematology, Oncology and Molecular Medicine, Istituto Superiore di Sanità, Rome, Italy

Paola Cassoni Department of Biomedical Sciences and Human Oncology, University of Turin, Turin, Italy

P. Corn Department of Genitourinary Medical Oncology–Research, The University of Texas M.D. Anderson Cancer Center, Houston, TX, USA

K. Edamura Department of Urology, Okayama University Graduate School of Medicine, Dentistry and Pharmaceutical Sciences, Okayama, Japan

Federica Felicetti Department of Hematology, Oncology and Molecular Medicine, Istituto Superiore di Sanità, Rome, Italy

A. Goltsov Department of Genitourinary Medical Oncology–Research, The University of Texas M.D. Anderson Cancer Center, Houston, TX, USA

Jorge Gutierrez-Pajares FONDAP Center for Molecular Studies of the Cell (CEMC), Universidad de Chile, Santiago, Chile

D. Kadmon Scott Department of Urology, Baylor College of Medicine, Houston, TX, USA

S. Kurosaka Department of Genitourinary Medical Oncology–Research, The University of Texas M.D. Anderson Cancer Center, Houston, TX, USA

L. Li Department of Genitourinary Medical Oncology–Research,
The University of Texas M.D. Anderson Cancer Center, Houston, TX, USA

Michael P. Lisanti Department of Stem Cell Biology & Regenerative Medicine,
Thomas Jefferson University, Philadelphia, PA, USA

C.J. Logothetis Department of Genitourinary Medical Oncology–Research,
The University of Texas M.D. Anderson Cancer Center, Houston, TX, USA

Isabelle Mercier Department of Stem Cell Biology & Regenerative Medicine,
Thomas Jefferson University, Philadelphia, PA, USA

Oeendree Mukherjee Department of Surgery, Jefferson Pancreas,
Biliary and Related Cancer Center, and Kimmel Cancer Center,
Thomas Jefferson University, Philadelphia, PA, USA

K. Naruishi Department of Pathophysiology–Periodontal Science,
Okayama University Graduate School of Medicine,
Dentistry and Pharmaceutical Sciences, Okayama, Japan

S. Park Department of Genitourinary Medical Oncology–Research,
The University of Texas M.D. Anderson Cancer Center, Houston, TX, USA

Isabella Parolini Department of Hematology, Oncology and Molecular
Medicine, Istituto Superiore di Sanità, Rome, Italy

Andrew F.G. Quest FONDAP Center for Molecular Studies
of the Cell (CEMC), Universidad de Chile, Santiago, Chile

C. Ren Department of Genitourinary Medical Oncology–Research,
The University of Texas M.D. Anderson Cancer Center, Houston, TX, USA

Nathan G. Richards Department of Surgery, Jefferson Pancreas,
Biliary and Related Cancer Center, and Kimmel Cancer Center,
Thomas Jefferson University, Philadelphia, PA, USA

David W. Rittenhouse Department of Surgery, Jefferson Pancreas,
Biliary and Related Cancer Center, and Kimmel Cancer Center,
Thomas Jefferson University, Philadelphia, PA, USA

Diego A. Rodriguez FONDAP Center for Molecular Studies
of the Cell (CEMC), Universidad de Chile, Santiago, Chile

Massimo Sargiacomo Department of Hematology, Oncology and Molecular
Medicine, Istituto Superiore di Sanità, Rome, Italy

Rebecca Senetta Department of Biomedical Sciences and Human Oncology,
University of Turin, Turin, Italy

Grzegorz Sowa Department of Medical Pharmacology and Physiology,
University of Missouri, Columbia, MO, USA

Ken-ichi Tabata Department of Urology, Kitasato School of Medicine, Tokyo, Japan

S.A. Tahir Department of Genitourinary Medical Oncology–Research, The University of Texas M.D. Anderson Cancer Center, Houston, TX, USA

R. Tanimoto Department of Genitourinary Medical Oncology–Research, The University of Texas M.D. Anderson Cancer Center, Houston, TX, USA

Julio C. Tapia FONDAP Center for Molecular Studies of the Cell (CEMC), Universidad de Chile, Santiago, Chile

T.C. Thompson Department of Genitourinary Medical Oncology–Research, The University of Texas M.D. Anderson Cancer Center, Houston, TX, USA

Vicente A. Torres FONDAP Center for Molecular Studies of the Cell (CEMC), Universidad de Chile, Santiago, Chile

P. Troncoso Department of Pathology, The University of Texas M.D. Anderson Cancer Center, Houston, TX, USA

M. Watanabe Department of Urology, Okayama University Graduate School of Medicine, Dentistry and Pharmaceutical Sciences, Okayama, Japan

Agnieszka K. Witkiewicz Department of Surgery, Jefferson Pancreas, Biliary and Related Cancer Center, and Kimmel Cancer Center, Thomas Jefferson University, Philadelphia, PA, USA

Department of Pathology, Thomas Jefferson University, Philadelphia, PA, USA

G. Yang Department of Genitourinary Medical Oncology–Research, The University of Texas M.D. Anderson Cancer Center, Houston, TX, USA

Charles J. Yeo Department of Surgery, Jefferson Pancreas, Biliary and Related Cancer Center, and Kimmel Cancer Center, Thomas Jefferson University, Philadelphia, PA, USA

Chapter 1
Local and Distant Effects of Caveolin-1 on Prostate Cancer Progression

T.C. Thompson, S.A. Tahir, L. Li, M. Watanabe, K. Naruishi, G. Yang, Ken-ichi Tabata, S. Kurosaka, K. Edamura, R. Tanimoto, P. Corn, D. Kadmon, C.J. Logothetis, P. Troncoso, C. Ren, A. Goltsov, and S. Park

Introduction

Although the mortality rates for specific cancers have declined modestly in recent years, overall, cancer remains the second leading cause of death, behind heart disease, in the entire population and is the leading cause of death for people in the United States between 60 and 79 years old. Estimates were that there would be 291,610 newly diagnosed cancers of the genitourinary (GU) tract in men and 46,840 deaths caused by those cancers in 2009; prostate cancer (PCa) alone would account for 66% of the new cases of GU cancer and 60% of cancer-related deaths in men [39]. PCa is androgen sensitive, and hormone therapy, mainly achieved by androgen deprivation, is one of the main treatment modalities in the clinical management of

T.C. Thompson (✉) • S.A. Tahir • L. Li • G. Yang • S. Kurosaka • R. Tanimoto • P. Corn
• C. J. Logothetis • C. Ren • A. Goltsov • S. Park
Department of Genitourinary Medical Oncology–Research, The University of Texas
M.D. Anderson Cancer Center, 1515 Holcombe Boulevard, Houston, TX 77030, USA
e-mail: timthomp@mdanderson.org

M. Watanabe • K. Edamura
Department of Urology, Okayama University Graduate School of Medicine,
Dentistry and Pharmaceutical Sciences, Okayama, Japan

K. Naruishi
Department of Pathophysiology–Periodontal Science, Okayama University Graduate School
of Medicine, Dentistry and Pharmaceutical Sciences, Okayama, Japan

K.-i. Tabata
Department of Urology, Kitasato School of Medicine, Tokyo, Japan

D. Kadmon
Scott Department of Urology,Baylor College of Medicine, Houston, TX, USA

P. Troncoso
Department of Pathology, The University of Texas M.D. Anderson Cancer Center,
Houston, TX, USA

I. Mercier et al. (eds.), *Caveolins in Cancer Pathogenesis, Prevention and Therapy*,
Current Cancer Research, DOI 10.1007/978-1-4614-1001-0_1,
© Springer Science+Business Media, LLC 2012

advanced PCa. However, this treatment is only palliative and has numerous side effects [56]. Recent clinical studies also indicate that docetaxel chemotherapy provides modest survival benefits in castrate-resistant PCa (CRPC) [66]. The development of therapies for metastatic PCa is the most significant challenge today in translational PCa research. Although metastatic PCa is a multifocal disease, bone is the principal organ involved by metastases. It is critically important to gain increased understanding of the mechanisms that underlie the development and progression of PCa to facilitate the development of biomarkers and novel therapeutic strategies to control this devastating malignancy.

Caveolin-1 (Cav-1) is a major structural component of the caveolae, which are specialized plasma membrane invaginations that are involved in multiple cellular processes, such as molecular transport, cell adhesion, and signal transduction [78, 84]. Cav-1 is expressed at relatively high levels in differentiated smooth muscle cells, pneumonocytes, chondrocytes, endothelial cells, adipocytes, and osteoblasts, in which it is associated with the acquisition and maintenance of specialized cell functions [29, 71, 80, 81]. Cav-1 exerts various biological functions through protein–protein interactions. Specific proteins, such as receptor tyrosine kinases, serine/threonine kinases, phospholipases, G protein-coupled receptors, and Src family kinases, are localized in lipid rafts and caveolar membranes, where they interact with Cav-1 through the Cav-1 scaffolding domain (CSD). CSD-mediated activities result in the generation of platforms for compartmentalization of discrete signaling events [64, 76].

The role of Cav-1 in tumorigenesis is complex and depends on the cell type and biological context. Under some conditions, Cav-1 may suppress tumorigenesis [103]. However, Cav-1 is associated with and contributes to malignant progression of multiple malignancies, including PCa [77, 93, 103]. Although the regulation of Cav-1 expression is complex, previous studies showed that Cav-1 expression is stimulated by testosterone and by multiple growth factors that are known to promote the development and progression of PCa [50, 52]. Cav-1 overexpression leads to promiscuous binding of Cav-1 to multiple signaling molecules in the cancer tyrosine-kinase regulatory network, including vascular endothelial growth factor receptor 2 (VEGFR2), platelet-derived growth factor receptor α/β (PDGFRα/β), Src, protein phosphatase 1/protein phosphatase 2A (PP1/PP2A) (negative regulator of Akt), and Phospholipase C γ1 (PLCγ1) through CSD–CSD binding-site interactions [51, 87]. These interactions increase PCa cell survival [51]. In addition, Cav-1 overexpression in PCa cells leads to Akt-mediated up-regulation of multiple cancer-promoting growth factors, including VEGF, transforming growth factor β1 (TGF-β1), and fibroblast growth factor 2 (FGF2) [50].

A critically important characteristic of many androgen-insensitive PCa cell lines is secretion of biologically active Cav-1 protein. PCa cell-derived secreted Cav-1 can promote PCa-cell viability through antiapoptotic activities and clonal growth in vitro, similar to those observed following enforced expression of Cav-1 within the cells [5, 51, 89, 104]. A recent study showed that recombinant Cav-1 protein is taken up by PCa cells and endothelial cells in vitro and that recombinant Cav-1 increases angiogenic activities both in vitro and in vivo by activating Akt- and/or nitric oxide synthase (NOS)-mediated signaling [90]. Cav-1-stimulated autocrine and paracrine engagement of the local tumor microenvironment involve but are not likely to be limited to the pro-angiogenic activities previously documented. It is important to note that significantly higher serum Cav-1 levels have been documented in men with PCa cancer than in men with benign prostatic hyperplasia [88] and in patients with elevated risk of cancer recurrence after radical prostatectomy [86].

Similar to the local effects of tumor cell-derived secreted Cav-1, serum Cav-1 can promote metastasis at distant sites [96]. Therefore, the pervasive effects of intracellular and secreted Cav-1 constitute positive-feedback loop that promotes PCa progression through unprecedented effects on the tumor microenvironment and metastatic environment. This chapter is a brief discussion of the complex and context-dependent activities of Cav-1 and delineation of the oncogenic functions of Cav-1 in PCa.

Aberrant Cav-1 Expression: Complexity and Context

Genetically engineered mouse models have proved invaluable for gaining an understanding of gene function and gaining insight into the role of specific proteins in human disease. Three independent groups of investigators have reported generation of Cav-1-knockout mice [8, 21, 70]. In all cases, $Cav-1^{-/-}$ mice were reported to be viable with no obvious abnormalities. However, further analysis revealed multiple abnormalities in cardiovascular, pulmonary, and urogenital tissues [13, 37, 65]. It is interesting that many of the functional abnormalities that were documented in studies of $Cav-1^{-/-}$ mice involved growth-related disorders in stromal cells that normally have high levels of Cav-1. A recent analysis of $Cav-1^{-/-}$ mice revealed stromal cell hyperplasias that could be interpreted as incomplete differentiation related to lack of Cav-1 [107]. In many organs in which loss of Cav-1 led to disorganized and/or hyperplastic stroma, growth and/or differentiation abnormalities were also observed in adjacent epithelial cells that normally express low to nondetectable levels of Cav-1. It was proposed that loss of Cav-1 function in stromal cells of various organs directly leads to a disorganized stromal compartment that, in turn, indirectly promotes abnormal growth and differentiation of adjacent epithelium.

Although the absence of Cav-1 has not been reported to increase the incidence of spontaneous malignancies, more hyperplastic lesions and tumors were observed in the skin of $Cav-1^{-/-}$ mice than in that of wild-type mice after application of dimethylbenzanthracene [9]. Further studies showed that loss of $Cav-1$ gene expression can accelerate the development of hyperplastic and dysplastic mammary lesions and enhance tumorgenesis and metastasis in cancer-prone genetically engineered mice [100, 102]. These results were consistent with those of previous studies, which showed that targeted down-regulation of Cav-1 increases tumorigenicity in NIH-3T3 mouse fibroblasts [25] and that enforced expression of Cav-1 suppresses the growth of fibroblasts and specific human breast cancer cell lines with myoepithelial cell features in vitro [48]. These and other study results led to the notion that $Cav-1$ is a tumor-suppressor gene [103].

In accordance with that notion, some reports have documented down-regulation of Cav-1 in various malignant human tissues, including osteosarcomas [7], fibrosarcomas [98], colon cancer [6], follicular thyroid cancer [1], ovarian cancer [17, 98], mucoepidermoid carcinoma of the salivary gland [79], lung adenocarcinoma [46, 99], and relatively small, estrogen receptor–positive breast cancer [73]. Numerous studies have not revealed any inactivating *Cav-1* mutations in tumors with Cav-1 down-regulation, but the recent identification of a dominant-negative mutation, a proline-to-leucine substitution at position 132 in human breast cancer tissues, may lead to further information about tumor-suppressor functions of Cav-1 [31]. Although there is not a perfect correlation, it is remarkable that many of these malignancies are of stromal cell origin. A recent novel and somewhat surprising observation is the reduction of Cav-1 levels in human cancer-associated fibroblasts from breast cancers and PCa [20, 60].

In contrast to studies of *Cav-1$^{-/-}$* that revealed its potential tumor-suppressor activities, recently published study results showed that *Cav-1$^{-/-}$* TRAMP (transgenic mouse prostate) mice demonstrate significantly fewer primary tumors and lesions than *Cav-1$^{+/+}$* TRAMP mice do [101]. Additional studies showed that transgenic mice with targeted overexpression of Cav-1 in prostatic epithelial cells using the short probasin (PB) promoter (i.e., PBcav-1 mice) demonstrated prostatic hyperplasia [96]. In addition, secreted Cav-1 from prostatic epithelial cells in PBcav-1 mice created a local microenvironment that permitted tumor growth and increased serum Cav-1 that was associated with increased experimental PCa lung metastasis activities. These results are consistent with those of numerous studies that have documented Cav-1 overexpression in PCa tissues [75, 105, 108, 109] and other malignancies, including esophageal squamous carcinoma [34, 45], oral carcinoma [35], papillary carcinoma of the thyroid [38], pancreatic cancer [85, 91], renal carcinoma [10, 33, 40], bladder cancer [68, 74], metastatic lung cancer [32], squamous carcinoma of the lung [110], Ewing sarcoma [94], and basal-like breast carcinomas [23, 27].

Although Cav-1 expression is complex, a substantial body of work now clearly indicates that it can demonstrate either growth-suppressive or oncogenic properties, depending on the type of malignant cell. This dichotomy will ultimately be defined at the molecular level through precise signaling analysis in well-controlled experiments and validation in clinical and pathologic studies. One of the clearest examples of a malignancy in which Cav-1 promotes tumor progression is PCa. Studies of PCa have provided insight into the underlying mechanisms of Cav-1-mediated oncogenic activities.

Overexpression of Cav-1 in Prostate Cancer

In previous studies, we reported greater Cav-1 immunostaining in human PCa cells than in adjacent normal prostatic epithelial cells, which express low to undetectable levels of Cav-1 [108, 109]. We further showed that increased Cav-1 immunostaining had independent prognostic potential in men undergoing radical prostatectomy [109].

These results were supported by two subsequent independent reports that also immunohistochemically evaluated PCa tissue and yielded similar conclusions [30, 44]. An important common observation from the cases examined in these studies is that immunostaining of Cav-1 in localized PCa is focal and that it is expressed in only a relatively small percentage of PCa cells. These results also showed that the presence of Cav-1 correlated positively with Gleason grade, an important suggestion that even though it is focally expressed, Cav-1 is a biomarker for clinically aggressive disease.

The molecular basis for the initiation of Cav-1 expression in PCa and other malignancies is not clear. The *Cav-1* and *Cav-2* genes are colocalized at 7q31.1, a highly conserved region that encompasses a known fragile site that is deleted, associated with loss of heterozygosity, or amplified in various human cancers, including PCa [13, 24, 63, 103]. Although some investigators have used these data to support a case for both loss and gain of Cav-1 expression, no convincing data specifically correlate genetic alterations at this site with changes in Cav-1 expression for PCa [4, 36]. The Cav-1 gene promoter has multiple CpG sites, and alterations in gene methylation have been demonstrated in PCa [15]. However, patterns of *Cav-1* gene methylation have not, thus far, provided a convincing argument for up-regulation of Cav-1 in PCa. It is interesting that the authors of a recent article suggest that loss of function for a tumor-suppressor microRNA (miR-205) may lead to up-regulation of Cav-1 in PCa [26].

Because many genetic alterations that occur in primary PCa have also been documented in premalignant disease such as high-grade prostatic intraepithelial neoplasia, it would be interesting to analyze Cav-1 in those premalignant lesions. Although it is focally expressed in primary PCa, it is important to note that Cav-1 is expressed in most metastatic cells [89]. This focal expression in primary PCa and significantly increased Cav-1 expression in associated metastases fits well with the notion that Cav-1 is more aligned with the criteria of a progression-related protein than with those of a protein that significantly affects localized tumor growth [92]. The idea of association of Cav-1 with clinically significant PCa is novel, and the prospect that Cav-1 expression may distinguish clinically significant PCa from clinically insignificant PCa is exciting [16].

Although the association between Cav-1 overexpression in PCa and aggressive, clinically significant disease has been found consistently in multiple studies, the relationship between Cav-1 overexpression and androgen sensitivity is less clear. Early studies showed that Cav-1 overexpression was inversely associated with androgen sensitivity and positively associated with tumor growth in mouse models of PCa [62]. The *Cav-1* gene is transcriptionally up-regulated in androgen-sensitive PCa cells, although the level of induction was modest [52]. In general, Cav-1 has been associated with the stimulatory effects of steroid receptors, including the androgen receptor, suggesting a point of convergence for further mechanistic studies [57, 69]. Overall, the available information on Cav-1 expression fits the hypothesis that PCa progression, even in the presence of normal levels of circulating testosterone, is coincidental with the development of androgen insensitivity. Certainly, the development of CRPC involves selection for unique malignant properties that allow PCa cells to metastasize in the presence of castrate levels of androgens. However, the emergence of CRPC does not preclude coselection of metastatic and androgen-insensitive PCa in men who have not undergone hormone therapy.

Cav-1-Mediated Oncogenic Activities in Prostate Cancer

The results of numerous studies that demonstrated overexpression of Cav-1-specific malignancies have led many investigators to attempt to identify Cav-1-related oncogenic pathways. Although Cav-1 activities impinge on various oncogenic pathways and can inhibit or activate these pathways, depending on the cell type and context [103], the results of multiple studies now indicate that Akt activation plays an important role in Cav-1-mediated oncogenic functions in PCa. The first demonstration of a direct association between Cav-1 expression and Akt indicated that the overexpression of Cav-1 increased binding to and inhibited the serine/threonine protein phosphatases PP1 and PP2A in human PCa cells. These interactions, which were likely mediated through the binding of Cav-1 to a CSD-binding site on PP1 and PP2A and inhibition of their activities, led to significantly increased levels of phospho-Akt and sustained activation of downstream oncogenic Akt targets [51]. Findings from a recent independent study supported this mechanism and further showed that the putative oncogene inhibitor of differentiation-1 (ID-1) induced Akt activation by promoting the binding activity of Cav-1 and PP2A [111]. It is important to consider that activation of Akt has been previously associated with PCa and is clearly one of the most important oncogenic activities that underlie progression of the disease [49].

A recent study further showed that alterations in Akt activities regulate the expression of fatty acid synthase, a putative metabolic oncogene, and its colocalization with Cav-1 in lipid rafts in PCa cells [18]. The same article reported that Src, an oncogenic tyrosine kinase, plays an important role in this process. It is notable that Cav-1 was initially identified as a v-Src substrate, P-Y14-Cav-1 [28]. Overall, these recent articles have suggested that an interactive and interdependent network of oncogenic proteins, including Cav-1, Akt, fatty acid synthase, and Src, plays an important role in PCa.

We recently demonstrated that in addition to promotion and maintenance of Akt activities, induction of Cav-1 expression led to enhanced tyrosine kinase signaling, which involved increased basal and VEGF-stimulated phosphorylation of VEGFR2, PLCγ1, and Akt, in PCa cells [87]. We have also shown that in PCa cells, a positive-feedback loop is established in which VEGF, TGF-β1, and FGF2 up-regulate Cav-1 expression, which in turn leads to increased levels of VEGF, TGF-β1, and FGF2 mRNA and protein, resulting in enhanced invasive activities (migration, motility) of PCa cells [50]. In the same study, we found that Akt-mediated Cav-1-enhanced mRNA stability is a major mechanism for the up-regulation of these cancer-promoting growth factors. In particular, Cav-1-mediated up-regulation and secretion of growth factors may lead to cell–cell signaling that involves the recruitment and functional activation of cancer-associated stromal cells (Fig. 1.1).

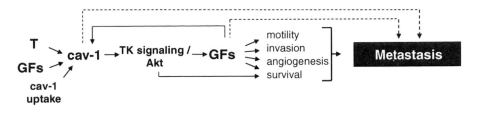

Fig. 1.1 Caveolin-1 (Cav-1)-growth factor (GF) positive-feedback system leads to prostate cancer (PCa) progression. GF-stimulated endogenous and secreted Cav-1 induces expression and secretion of GFs, which maintain Cav-1 expression and stimulate malignant activities both locally and at distant metastatic sites. *T*: Testosterone; *TK*: tyrosine kinase

These oncogenic protein networks appear to be important pathways through which Cav-1 promotes malignant activities in PCa. The results of a recent study showed that cellular levels of P-Y14-Cav-1 are critically associated with Rho/ROCK and Src-dependent regulation of tumor cell motility and invasion [41]. These results demonstrate that there are multiple pathways through which overexpression of Cav-1 may promote progression of PCa and other malignancies.

Secretion of Cav-1 by Prostate Cancer Cells

Cav-1, which is secreted by mouse and human PCa cell lines, promotes cancer cell survival in vitro [89]. These results were validated in independent studies and extended to include perineural cells in the PCa microenvironment [3, 5]. At the time these results were reported, those from a previous study had shown that Cav-1 was secreted by normal pancreatic acinar cells in vitro [54] but, to our knowledge, there were no previous reports of the secretion of Cav-1 by malignant cells.

These results raised the question about the mechanism responsible for Cav-1 secretion from cancer cells and whether this mechanism was specific to PCa cells or the PCa microenvironment. An intriguing article reported that Cav-1 was found in "prostasomes," which are vesicular organelles enriched with raft components, of PC-3 cells, suggesting that Cav-1 is secreted by PCa cells through a unique mechanism [55]. The results of a more recent study supported the concept that Cav-1 is secreted by PCa cells through a unique exosome–prostasome-mediated pathway [58]. More recently, Cav-1 was shown to be a major component of "oncosomes," i.e., membrane-derived microvesicles secreted by cancer cells. Oncosome formation was stimulated by epidermal growth factor receptor stimulation and by overexpression of membrane-targeted Akt in PCa cells. It was further demonstrated that "oncosomes" that were shed from PCa cells contained signal-transduction proteins, including Cav-1, that are capable of activating phospho-tyrosine and Akt-signaling pathways [19].

Additional studies are warranted to further characterize the specificity and mechanism(s) involved in Cav-1 secretion by PCa cells and potentially by specific stromal cells within the PCa microenvironment. It will also be important to further investigate the mechanism(s) underlying the release of microvesicles, i.e., "prostasomes" and/or "oncosomes," from PCa cells and their potential uptake by other cancer cells and PCa-associated stromal cells, vis-à-vis expression, secretion, and uptake of Cav-1.

Prostate Cancer-Derived Secreted Cav-1 Alters the Local Tumor Microenvironment

PCa is unique in its capacity to influence and become dependent on stromal cells that reside in the tumor microenvironment. Growth factors derived from PCa cells, including VEGF, TGF-β1, and multiple FGFs, are known to significantly affect, through autocrine and paracrine activities, the capacity of PCa cells to grow and metastasize [12, 47, 61, 72]. Various mechanisms are reportedly involved in the deregulation of these growth factors in cancer cells, including transcriptional regulation [42] and alteration of mRNA stability [11, 43, 82, 95].

We recently found, unexpectedly, that PCa-derived secreted Cav-1 is also capable of substantially altering the tumor microenvironment by stimulating angiogenesis. Specifically, Cav-1 is taken up by Cav-1-negative tumor cells and/or endothelial cells, leading to stimulation of specific angiogenic activities through the PI3K–Akt–eNOS signaling module [90]. This work followed a previous study that had found greater angiogenesis in Cav-1-positive PCa than in Cav-1-negative PCa and that also showed co-localization of Cav-1 with VEGFR2 in tumor-associated endothelial cells [106].

Recently we have extended these results in studies which demonstrated that treatment of PCa cells or endothelial cells with recombinant Cav-1 leads to induction of VEGF/VEGFR-mediated angiogenic signaling [87]. These angiogenic signaling activities likely play a central role in the positive-feedback loop that is established when VEGF, TGF-β1, and FGF2 up-regulate Cav-1 expression, which in turn leads to increased levels of VEGF, TGF-β1, and FGF2 mRNA and protein, resulting in enhanced invasive activities (migration, motility) of PCa cells [50]. It is notable that a common focal point of Cav-1 stimulated oncogenic signaling is activation of Akt. We have shown that Cav-1 can activate Akt through the binding of Cav-1 to a CSD-binding site on PP1 and PP2A and inhibition of their Akt-inhibitory activities [50]. We recently found that Akt-mediated Cav-1-enhanced mRNA stability is a major mechanism for the up-regulation of VEGF, TGF-β1, and FGF2 [50]. Clearly Akt activation is an important oncogenic target for endogenously expressed and secreted Cav-1 [50, 87, 90].

The combined action of PCa-derived secreted Cav-1 and its stimulation of growth factors and/or angiogenic cytokines could have a profound effect on the PCa microenvironment. Cav-1 uptake by and growth factor binding to tumor-associated stromal cells, including endothelial cells, could potentially result in structural modification of the preexisting signaling pathways through the interaction of Cav-1 with specific signaling molecules (Fig. 1.1).

Because many of the molecules involved in angiogenic signaling pathways possess CSD-binding sites, e.g., VEGFR2 and Src [14, 53, 64], these interactions are likely mediated in part through the CSD-binding site interface. To demonstrate the biologic effect of these activities, we recently showed that adult male PBcav-1 transgenic mice had significantly greater prostatic wet weight and a higher incidence of prostatic epithelial hyperplasia than did their nontransgenic littermates [96]. Prostatic tissues from the PBcav-1 transgenic mice, which also had greater Cav-1 secretory activities than did those from their nontransgenic littermates, also showed greater immunostaining for proliferative cell nuclear antigen and P-Akt, less nuclear p27^{Kip1} in hyperplastic lesions, and increased resistance to castration-induced prostate regression. An important note is that orthotopic prostatic injection of androgen-sensitive Cav-1-secreting RM-9 mouse PCa cells resulted in tumors that were significantly larger in PBcav-1 mice than they were in the nontransgenic littermates [96]. These results demonstrate that prostate cell-derived secreted Cav-1 can result in hyperplastic epithelial growth abnormalities and lead to a prostatic environment that permits PCa growth.

The expression and secretion of Cav-1 by PCa cells presents an opportunity for the development of Cav-1-based biomarkers for PCa. We previously developed an immunoassay for measuring serum Cav-1 levels and showed that the median serum Cav-1 level in men with clinically localized PCa was significantly higher than that in healthy control men (i.e., those with normal findings on digital rectal examination and serum prostate-specific antigen (PSA) levels of ≤1.5 ng mL^{-1} over a period of 2 years) and in men with clinical benign prostatic hyperplasia [88]. Further, in a larger population study in men with a serum PSA of >10 ng mL^{-1}, high levels of Cav-1 in serum prior to treatment were associated with a shorter time to biochemical recurrence (defined as a serum PSA level of ≥ 0.2 ng mL^{-1} on two consecutive measurements) [86]. High pretreatment serum Cav-1 levels were established using a cutoff determined by using the minimum P value method.

These initial clinical and basic laboratory study results, together with those of pathology-based tissue analysis, demonstrate the potential of serum Cav-1 as a prognostic biomarker for identification of men with clinically aggressive PCa. Specifically, the pretreatment serum Cav-1 concentration may be used to identify men with clinically significant PCa who are likely to experience rapid recurrence of the cancer following radical prostatectomy. Although further studies are necessary to validate these results, it is conceivable that serum Cav-1 analysis would contribute to the identification of a subset of men undergoing localized therapy for presumed localized disease who would benefit from neoadjuvant or adjuvant therapy, e.g., local radiotherapy, localized biologic therapy, androgen-deprivation therapy, and/or targeted systemic therapy [2, 22, 67, 83].

Prostate Cancer-Derived Secreted Cav-1 Alters Metastatic Tumor Microenvironment

Generation of the PBcav-1 transgenic mouse gave us the opportunity to test the potential role of prostate epithelial cell-derived secreted Cav-1 in PCa metastasis. We demonstrated that male PBcav-1 mice had significantly greater serum Cav-1 levels than did their nontransgenic littermates [96]. Tail-vein inoculation of RM-9 mouse PCa cells produced significantly more experimental lung metastases in male PBcav-1 than in their nontransgenic littermates and in male *Cav-1*$^{+/+}$ mice than in male *Cav-1*$^{-/-}$ mice [96]. Systemic treatment with anti-Cav-1 antibody dramatically reduced the number of experimental metastases, demonstrating prometastatic activities for PCa-derived secreted Cav-1 in this model system. These results further reveal the possibility that secreted Cav-1 is a therapeutic target for PCa. Because targeted systemic antibody therapy has been used successfully to treat specific malignancies [59, 97], the development of Cav-1-targeted antibody therapy should be further pursued as a potential therapy for PCa.

Summary

The initial observations that PCa cells overexpress Cav-1 and that Cav-1 is associated with clinically significant PCa have led to extensive basic laboratory and clinical studies of the role of Cav-1 in PCa and other malignancies. Although the molecular and cellular biology of Cav-1 is complex, the studies thus far have shown that the overexpression and secretion of Cav-1 leads to amplification of the tumor-promoting effects of Cav-1 through activation of endogenous oncogenic pathways and engagement of the tumor microenvironment. The remarkable capacity of Cav-1 to restructure and participate in PCa cell signaling and to stimulate expression of cancer-associated growth factors is a novel paradigm in oncogene research. Recent studies have extended our knowledge of the unique and unprecedented effects of PCa-derived secreted Cav-1 on the local and metastatic tumor microenvironments. According to study results that show Cav-1 as a component of "prostasomes" and/or "oncosomes," it is important to better understand the relationships between membrane-mediated and "free" Cav-1 release and uptake by other PCa cells and by PCa-associated stromal cells, including endothelial cells. The association between Cav-1 and clinically significant PCa is unique, and the prospect that Cav-1 expression may differentiate clinically significant from clinically insignificant PCa is exciting. By virtue of the capacity of PCa cells to secrete Cav-1, specific Cav-1-based biomarkers and therapeutic strategies have been proposed and tested. The initial results are promising and indicate that further studies may lead to clinically useful prognostic and therapeutic tools for PCa.

Acknowledgment This work was supported in part by National Institutes of Health grant R01 CA68814, P30 CA016672, and Department of Defense grant DAMD PC051247.

References

1. Aldred MA, Ginn-Pease ME, Morrison CD et al (2003) Caveolin-1 and caveolin-2, together with three bone morphogenetic protein-related genes, may encode novel tumor suppressors down-regulated in sporadic follicular thyroid carcinogenesis. Cancer Res 63(11):2864–2871
2. Ayala G, Satoh T, Li R et al (2006) Biological response determinants in HSV-tk + ganciclovir gene therapy for prostate cancer. Mol Ther 13(4):716–728

3. Ayala GE, Dai H, Tahir SA et al (2006) Stromal antiapoptotic paracrine loop in perineural invasion of prostatic carcinoma. Cancer Res 66(10):5159–5164

4. Bachmann N, Haeusler J, Luedeke M et al (2008) Expression changes of CAV1 and EZH2, located on 7q31 approximately q36, are rarely related to genomic alterations in primary prostate carcinoma. Cancer Genet Cytogenet 182(2):103–110

5. Bartz R, Zhou J, Hsieh JT et al (2008) Caveolin-1 secreting LNCaP cells induce tumor growth of caveolin-1 negative LNCaP cells in vivo. Int J Cancer 122(3):520–525

6. Bender FC, Reymond MA, Bron C et al (2000) Caveolin-1 levels are down-regulated in human colon tumors, and ectopic expression of caveolin-1 in colon carcinoma cell lines reduces cell tumorigenicity. Cancer Res 60(20):5870–5878

7. Cantiani L, Manara MC, Zucchini C et al (2007) Caveolin-1 reduces osteosarcoma metastases by inhibiting c-Src activity and met signaling. Cancer Res 67(16):7675–7685

8. Cao G, Yang G, Timme TL et al (2003) Disruption of the caveolin-1 gene impairs renal calcium reabsorption and leads to hypercalciuria and urolithiasis. Am J Pathol 162(4):1241–1248

9. Capozza F, Williams TM, Schubert W et al (2003) Absence of caveolin-1 sensitizes mouse skin to carcinogen-induced epidermal hyperplasia and tumor formation. Am J Pathol 162(6):2029–2039

10. Carrion R, Morgan BE, Tannenbaum M et al (2003) Caveolin expression in adult renal tumors. Urol Oncol 21(3):191–196

11. Cash J, Korchnak A, Gorman J et al (2007) VEGF transcription and mRNA stability are altered by WT1 not DDS(R384W) expression in LNCaP cells. Oncol Rep 17(6):1413–1419

12. Chung LW, Huang WC, Sung SY et al (2006) Stromal-epithelial interaction in prostate cancer progression. Clin Genitourin Cancer 5(2):162–170

13. Cohen AW, Hnasko R, Schubert W et al (2004) Role of caveolae and caveolins in health and disease. Physiol Rev 84(4):1341–1379

14. Couet J, Li S, Okamoto T et al (1997) Identification of peptide and protein ligands for the caveolin-scaffolding domain. Implications for the interaction of caveolin with caveolae-associated proteins. J Biol Chem 272(10):6525–6533

15. Cui J, Rohr LR, Swanson G et al (2001) Hypermethylation of the caveolin-1 gene promoter in prostate cancer. Prostate 46(3):249–256

16. Dall'era MA, Cooperberg MR, Chan JM et al (2008) Active surveillance for early-stage prostate cancer: review of the current literature. Cancer 112(8):1650–1659

17. Davidson B, Nesland JM, Goldberg I et al (2001) Caveolin-1 expression in advanced-stage ovarian carcinoma – a clinicopathologic study. Gynecol Oncol 81(2):166–171

18. Di Vizio D, Adam RM, Kim J et al (2008) Caveolin-1 interacts with a lipid raft-associated population of fatty acid synthase. Cell Cycle 7(14):2257–2267

19. Di Vizio D, Kim J, Hager MH et al (2009) Oncosome formation in prostate cancer: association with a region of frequent chromosomal deletion in metastatic disease. Cancer Res 69(13):5601–5609

20. Di Vizio D, Morello M, Sotgia F et al (2009) An absence of stromal caveolin-1 is associated with advanced prostate cancer, metastatic disease and epithelial Akt activation. Cell Cycle 8(15):2420–2424

21. Drab M, Verkade P, Elger M et al (2001) Loss of caveolae, vascular dysfunction, and pulmonary defects in caveolin-1 gene-disrupted mice. Science 293(5539):2449–2452

22. Efstathiou E, Troncoso P, Wen S et al (2007) Initial modulation of the tumor microenvironment accounts for thalidomide activity in prostate cancer. Clin Cancer Res 13(4):1224–1231

23. Elsheikh SE, Green AR, Rakha EA et al (2008) Caveolin 1 and caveolin 2 are associated with breast cancer basal-like and triple-negative immunophenotype. Br J Cancer 99(2):327–334

24. Engelman JA, Zhang XL, Lisanti MP (1998) Genes encoding human caveolin-1 and -2 are co-localized to the D7S522 locus (7q31.1), a known fragile site (FRA7G) that is frequently deleted in human cancers. FEBS Lett 436(3):403–410

25. Galbiati F, Volonte D, Engelman JA et al (1998) Targeted downregulation of caveolin-1 is sufficient to drive cell transformation and hyperactivate the p42/44 MAP kinase cascade. EMBO J 17(22):6633–6648

26. Gandellini P, Folini M, Longoni N et al (2009) miR-205 Exerts tumor-suppressive functions in human prostate through down-regulation of protein kinase Cepsilon. Cancer Res 69(6):2287–2295

27. Garcia S, Dales JP, Charafe-Jauffret E et al (2007) Poor prognosis in breast carcinomas correlates with increased expression of targetable CD146 and c-Met and with proteomic basal-like phenotype. Hum Pathol 38(6):830–841

28. Glenney JR Jr, Zokas L (1989) Novel tyrosine kinase substrates from Rous sarcoma virus-transformed cells are present in the membrane skeleton. J Cell Biol 108(6):2401–2408

29. Goetz JG, Lajoie P, Wiseman SM et al (2008) Caveolin-1 in tumor progression: the good, the bad and the ugly. Cancer Metastasis Rev 27(4):715–735

30. Goto T, Nguyen BP, Nakano M et al (2008) Utility of Bcl-2, P53, Ki-67, and caveolin-1 immunostaining in the prediction of biochemical failure after radical prostatectomy in a Japanese population. Urology 72(1):167–171

31. Hayashi K, Matsuda S, Machida K et al (2001) Invasion activating caveolin-1 mutation in human schirrhous breast cancer. Cancer Res 61:2361–2364

32. Ho CC, Huang PH, Huang HY et al (2002) Up-regulated caveolin-1 accentuates the metastasis capability of lung adenocarcinoma by inducing filopodia formation. Am J Pathol 161(5):1647–1656

33. Horiguchi A, Asano T, Asakuma J et al (2004) Impact of caveolin-1 expression on clinico-pathological parameters in renal cell carcinoma. J Urol 172(2):718–722

34. Hu YC, Lam KY, Law S et al (2001) Profiling of differentially expressed cancer-related genes in esophageal squamous cell carcinoma (ESCC) using human cancer cDNA arrays: overexpression of oncogene MET correlates with tumor differentiation in ESCC. Clin Cancer Res 7(11):3519–3525

35. Hung KF, Lin SC, Liu CJ et al (2003) The biphasic differential expression of the cellular membrane protein, caveolin-1, in oral carcinogenesis. J Oral Pathol Med 32(8):461–467

36. Hurlstone AF, Reid G, Reeves JR et al (1999) Analysis of the CAVEOLIN-1 gene at human chromosome 7q31.1 in primary tumours and tumour-derived cell lines. Oncogene 18(10):1881–1890

37. Insel PA, Patel HH (2007) Do studies in caveolin-knockouts teach us about physiology and pharmacology or instead, the ways mice compensate for 'lost proteins'? Br J Pharmacol 150(3):251–254

38. Ito Y, Yoshida H, Nakano K et al (2002) Caveolin-1 overexpression is an early event in the progression of papillary carcinoma of the thyroid. Br J Cancer 86(6):912–916

39. Jemal A, Siegel R, Ward E et al (2009) Cancer statistics, 2009. CA Cancer J Clin 59(4):225–249

40. Joo HJ, Oh DK, Kim YS et al (2004) Increased expression of caveolin-1 and microvessel density correlates with metastasis and poor prognosis in clear cell renal cell carcinoma. BJU Int 93(3):291–296

41. Joshi B, Strugnell SS, Goetz JG et al (2008) Phosphorylated caveolin-1 regulates Rho/ROCK-dependent focal adhesion dynamics and tumor cell migration and invasion. Cancer Res 68(20):8210–8220

42. Josko J, Mazurek M (2004) Transcription factors having impact on vascular endothelial growth factor VEGF gene expression in angiogenesis. Med Sci Monit 10(4):RA89–RA98

43. Kanies CL, Smith JJ, Kis C et al (2008) Oncogenic Ras and transforming growth factor-beta synergistically regulate AU-rich element-containing mRNAs during epithelial to mesenchymal transition. Mol Cancer Res 6(7):1124–1136

44. Karam JA, Lotan Y, Roehrborn CG et al (2007) Caveolin-1 overexpression is associated with aggressive prostate cancer recurrence. Prostate 67(6):614–622

45. Kato K, Hida Y, Miyamoto M et al (2002) Overexpression of caveolin-1 in esophageal squamous cell carcinoma correlates with lymph node metastasis and pathologic stage. Cancer 94(4):929–933

46. Kato T, Miyamoto M, Kato K et al (2004) Difference of caveolin-1 expression pattern in human lung neoplastic tissue. Atypical adenomatous hyperplasia, adenocarcinoma and squamous cell carcinoma. Cancer Lett 214(1):121–128

47. Kwabi-Addo B, Ozen M, Ittmann M (2004) The role of fibroblast growth factors and their receptors in prostate cancer. Endocr Relat Cancer 11(4):709–724
48. Lee SW, Reimer CL, Oh P et al (1998) Tumor cell growth inhibition by caveolin re-expression in human breast cancer cells. Oncogene 16(11):1391–1397
49. Li L, Ittmann MM, Ayala G et al (2005) The emerging role of the PI3-K-Akt pathway in prostate cancer progression. Prostate Cancer Prostatic Dis 8(2):108–118
50. Li L, Ren C, Yang G et al (2009) Caveolin-1 promotes autoregulatory, Akt-mediated induction of cancer-promoting growth factors in prostate cancer cells. Mol Cancer Res 7(11): 1781–1791
51. Li L, Ren CH, Tahir SA et al (2003) Caveolin-1 maintains activated Akt in prostate cancer cells through scaffolding domain binding site interactions with and inhibition of serine/threonine protein phosphatases PP1 and PP2A. Mol Cell Biol 23(24):9389–9404
52. Li L, Yang G, Ebara S et al (2001) Caveolin-1 mediates testosterone-stimulated survival/ clonal growth and promotes metastatic activities in prostate cancer cells. Cancer Res 61(11): 4386–4392
53. Li S, Couet J, Lisanti MP (1996) Src tyrosine kinases, Galpha subunits, and H-Ras share a common membrane-anchored scaffolding protein, caveolin. Caveolin binding negatively regulates the auto-activation of Src tyrosine kinases. J Biol Chem 271(46):29182–29190
54. Liu P, Li WP, Machleidt T et al (1999) Identification of caveolin-1 in lipoprotein particles secreted by exocrine cells. Nat Cell Biol 1(6):369–375
55. Llorente A, de Marco MC, Alonso MA (2004) Caveolin-1 and MAL are located on prostasomes secreted by the prostate cancer PC-3 cell line. J Cell Sci 117(pt 22):5343–5351
56. Loblaw DA, Virgo KS, Nam R et al (2007) Initial hormonal management of androgen-sensitive metastatic, recurrent, or progressive prostate cancer: 2006 update of an American Society of Clinical Oncology practice guideline. J Clin Oncol 25(12):1596–1605
57. Lu ML, Schneider MC, Zheng Y et al (2001) Caveolin-1 interacts with androgen receptor. A positive modulator of androgen receptor mediated transactivation. J Biol Chem 276(16): 13442–13451
58. Lu Q, Zhang J, Allison R et al (2009) Identification of extracellular delta-catenin accumulation for prostate cancer detection. Prostate 69(4):411–418
59. Ma WW, Adjei AA (2009) Novel agents on the horizon for cancer therapy. CA Cancer J Clin 59(2):111–137
60. Mercier I, Casimiro MC, Wang C et al (2008) Human breast cancer-associated fibroblasts (CAFs) show caveolin-1 downregulation and RB tumor suppressor functional inactivation: implications for the response to hormonal therapy. Cancer Biol Ther 7(8):1212–1225
61. Morrissey C, Vessella RL (2007) The role of tumor microenvironment in prostate cancer bone metastasis. J Cell Biochem 101(4):873–886
62. Nasu Y, Timme TL, Yang G et al (1998) Suppression of caveolin expression induces androgen sensitivity in metastatic androgen-insensitive mouse prostate cancer cells [see comments]. Nat Med 4(9):1062–1064
63. Nupponen NN, Kakkola L, Koivisto P et al (1998) Genetic alterations in hormone-refractory recurrent prostate carcinomas. Am J Pathol 153(1):141–148
64. Okamoto T, Schlegel A, Scherer PE et al (1998) Caveolins, a family of scaffolding proteins for organizing "preassembled signaling complexes" at the plasma membrane. J Biol Chem 273(10):5419–5422
65. Patel HH, Murray F, Insel PA (2008) Caveolae as organizers of pharmacologically relevant signal transduction molecules. Annu Rev Pharmacol Toxicol 48:359–391
66. Petrylak DP, Tangen CM, Hussain MH et al (2004) Docetaxel and estramustine compared with mitoxantrone and prednisone for advanced refractory prostate cancer. N Engl J Med 351(15):1513–1520
67. Pisters LL, Pettaway CA, Troncoso P et al (2004) Evidence that transfer of functional p53 protein results in increased apoptosis in prostate cancer. Clin Cancer Res 10(8):2587–2593
68. Rajjayabun PH, Garg S, Durkan GC et al (2001) Caveolin-1 expression is associated with high-grade bladder cancer. Urology 58(5):811–814

69. Razandi M, Alton G, Pedram A et al (2003) Identification of a structural determinant necessary for the localization and function of estrogen receptor alpha at the plasma membrane. Mol Cell Biol 23(5):1633–1646
70. Razani B, Engelman JA, Wang XB et al (2001) Caveolin-1 null mice are viable but show evidence of hyperproliferative and vascular abnormalities. J Biol Chem 276(41):38121–38138
71. Razani B, Lisanti MP (2001) Caveolin-deficient mice: insights into caveolar function human disease. J Clin Invest 108(11):1553–1561
72. Reynolds AR, Kyprianou N (2006) Growth factor signalling in prostatic growth: significance in tumour development and therapeutic targeting. Br J Pharmacol 147(suppl 2):S144–S152
73. Sagara Y, Mimori K, Yoshinaga K et al (2004) Clinical significance of caveolin-1, caveolin-2 and HER2/neu mRNA expression in human breast cancer. Br J Cancer 91(5):959–965
74. Sanchez-Carbayo M, Socci ND, Charytonowicz E et al (2002) Molecular profiling of bladder cancer using cDNA microarrays: defining histogenesis and biological phenotypes. Cancer Res 62(23):6973–6980
75. Satoh T, Yang G, Egawa S et al (2003) Caveolin-1 expression is a predictor of recurrence-free survival in pT2N0 prostate carcinoma diagnosed in Japanese patients. Cancer 97(5):1225–1233
76. Schlegel A, Schwab RB, Scherer PE et al (1999) A role for the caveolin scaffolding domain in mediating the membrane attachment of caveolin-1. The caveolin scaffolding domain is both necessary and sufficient for membrane binding in vitro. J Biol Chem 274(32):22660–22667
77. Shatz M, Liscovitch M (2008) Caveolin-1: a tumor-promoting role in human cancer. Int J Radiat Biol 84(3):177–189
78. Shaul PW, Anderson RG (1998) Role of plasmalemmal caveolae in signal transduction. Am J Physiol 275(5 pt 1):L843–L851
79. Shi L, Chen XM, Wang L et al (2007) Expression of caveolin-1 in mucoepidermoid carcinoma of the salivary glands: correlation with vascular endothelial growth factor, microvessel density, and clinical outcome. Cancer 109(8):1523–1531
80. Smart EJ, Graf GA, McNiven MA et al (1999) Caveolins, liquid-ordered domains, and signal transduction. Mol Cell Biol 19(11):7289–7304
81. Solomon KR, Danciu TE, Adolphson LD et al (2000) Caveolin-enriched membrane signaling complexes in human and murine osteoblasts. J Bone Miner Res 15(12):2380–2390
82. Song QH, Klepeis VE, Nugent MA et al (2002) TGF-beta1 regulates TGF-beta1 and FGF-2 mRNA expression during fibroblast wound healing. Mol Pathol 55(3):164–176
83. Sonpavde G, Chi KN, Powles T et al (2007) Neoadjuvant therapy followed by prostatectomy for clinically localized prostate cancer. Cancer 110(12):2628–2639
84. Sternberg PW, Schmid SL (1999) Caveolin, cholesterol and Ras signalling. Nat Cell Biol 1(2):E35–E37
85. Suzuoki M, Miyamoto M, Kato K et al (2002) Impact of caveolin-1 expression on prognosis of pancreatic ductal adenocarcinoma. Br J Cancer 87(10):1140–1144
86. Tahir SA, Frolov A, Hayes TG, Mims MP, Miles BJ, Lerner SP, Wheeler TM, Ayala G, Thompson TC, Kadmon D (2006) Preoperative serum caveolin-1 as a prognostic marker for recurrence in a radical prostatectomy cohort. Clin Cancer Res 12(16):4872–4875
87. Tahir SA, Park S, Thompson TC (2009) Caveolin-1 regulates VEGF-stimulated angiogenic activities in prostate cancer and endothelial cells. Cancer Biol Ther 8(23):2286–2296
88. Tahir SA, Ren C, Timme TL et al (2003) Development of an immunoassay for serum caveolin-1: a novel biomarker for prostate cancer. Clin Cancer Res 9(10 pt 1):3653–3659
89. Tahir SA, Yang G, Ebara S et al (2001) Secreted caveolin-1 stimulates cell survival/clonal growth and contributes to metastasis in androgen-insensitive prostate cancer. Cancer Res 61(10):3882–3885
90. Tahir SA, Yang G, Goltsov AA et al (2008) Tumor cell-secreted caveolin-1 has proangiogenic activities in prostate cancer. Cancer Res 68(3):731–739
91. Terris B, Blaveri E, Crnogorac-Jurcevic T et al (2002) Characterization of gene expression profiles in intraductal papillary-mucinous tumors of the pancreas. Am J Pathol 160(5):1745–1754
92. Thompson TC, Park SH, Timme TL et al (1995) Loss of p53 function leads to metastasis in ras + myc-initiated mouse prostate cancer. Oncogene 10(5):869–879

93. Thompson TC, Tahir SA, Li L et al (2010) The role of caveolin-1 in prostate cancer: clinical implications. Prostate Cancer Prostatic Dis 13(1):6–11
94. Tirado OM, Mateo-Lozano S, Villar J et al (2006) Caveolin-1 (CAV1) is a target of EWS/FLI-1 and a key determinant of the oncogenic phenotype and tumorigenicity of Ewing's sarcoma cells. Cancer Res 66(20):9937–9947
95. Touriol C, Morillon A, Gensac MC et al (1999) Expression of human fibroblast growth factor 2 mRNA is post-transcriptionally controlled by a unique destabilizing element present in the 3′-untranslated region between alternative polyadenylation sites. J Biol Chem 274(30):21402–21408
96. Watanabe M, Yang G, Cao G et al (2009) Functional analysis of secreted caveolin-1 in mouse models of prostate cancer progression. Mol Cancer Res 7(9):1446–1455
97. Weiner GJ (2007) Monoclonal antibody mechanisms of action in cancer. Immunol Res 39(1–3):271–278
98. Wiechen K, Sers C, Agoulnik A et al (2001) Down-regulation of caveolin-1, a candidate tumor suppressor gene, in sarcomas. Am J Pathol 158(3):833–839
99. Wikman H, Seppanen JK, Sarhadi VK et al (2004) Caveolins as tumour markers in lung cancer detected by combined use of cDNA and tissue microarrays. J Pathol 203(1):584–593
100. Williams TM, Cheung MW, Park DS et al (2003) Loss of caveolin-1 gene expression accelerates the development of dysplastic mammary lesions in tumor-prone transgenic mice. Mol Biol Cell 14(3):1027–1042
101. Williams TM, Hassan GS, Li J et al (2005) Caveolin-1 promotes tumor progression in an autochthonous mouse model of prostate cancer: genetic ablation of Cav-1 delays advanced prostate tumor development in TRAMP mice. J Biol Chem 10:1074
102. Williams TM, Lee H, Cheung MW et al (2004) Combined loss of INK4a and caveolin-1 synergistically enhances cell proliferation and oncogene-induced tumorigenesis: role of INK4a/CAV-1 in mammary epithelial cell hyperplasia. J Biol Chem 279(23):24745–24756
103. Williams TM, Lisanti MP (2005) Caveolin-1 in oncogenic transformation, cancer, and metastasis. Am J Physiol Cell Physiol 288(3):C494–C506
104. Wu D, Foreman TL, Gregory CW et al (2002) Protein kinase cepsilon has the potential to advance the recurrence of human prostate cancer. Cancer Res 62(8):2423–2429
105. Yang G, Addai J, Ittmann M et al (2000) Elevated caveolin-1 levels in African-American versus white-American prostate cancer. Clin Cancer Res 6(9):3430–3433
106. Yang G, Addai J, Wheeler TM et al (2007) Correlative evidence that prostate cancer cell-derived caveolin-1 mediates angiogenesis. Hum Pathol 38(11):1688–1695
107. Yang G, Timme TL, Naruishi K et al (2008) Mice with cav-1 gene disruption have benign stromal lesions and compromised epithelial differentiation. Exp Mol Pathol 84(2):131–140
108. Yang G, Truong LD, Timme TL et al (1998) Elevated expression of caveolin is associated with prostate and breast cancer. Clin Cancer Res 4(8):1873–1880
109. Yang G, Truong LD, Wheeler TM et al (1999) Caveolin-1 expression in clinically confined human prostate cancer: a novel prognostic marker. Cancer Res 59(22):5719–5723
110. Yoo SH, Park YS, Kim HR et al (2003) Expression of caveolin-1 is associated with poor prognosis of patients with squamous cell carcinoma of the lung. Lung Cancer 42(2):195–202
111. Zhang X, Ling MT, Wang Q et al (2007) Identification of a novel inhibitor of differentiation-1 (ID-1) binding partner, caveolin-1, and its role in epithelial-mesenchymal transition and resistance to apoptosis in prostate cancer cells. J Biol Chem 282(46):33284–33294

Chapter 2
Caveolin-1 in Colon Cancer: The Flexible Connection to Wnt Signaling

Andrew F.G. Quest, Vicente A. Torres, Diego A. Rodriguez,
Jorge Gutierrez-Pajares, and Julio C. Tapia

Abbreviations

AA	Arachidonic acid
APC	Adenomatous polyposis coli
CK1	Casein kinase 1
CK2	Casein kinase 2
COX-2	Cyclooxygenase-2
CSD	Caveolin scaffolding domain
Dvl	Disheveled
FAP	Familial adenomatous polyposis
GSK3β	Glycogen synthase kinase 3β
HNPCC	Hereditary non-polyposis colorectal cancer
IAP	Inhibitor of apoptosis
LRP	Low-density lipoprotein receptor-related protein
MDR	Multidrug resistance
NSAIDs	Nonsteroidal anti-inflammatory drugs
PCP	Planar cell polarity
PGE_2	Prostaglandin E_2
PGH_2	Prostaglandin H_2
SCF	Skp1-Cul1-F-box-protein
Tcf/Lef	T cell factor/lymphoid enhancer binding factor
βTrCP	β-Transducin repeat containing protein

A.F.G. Quest (✉) • V.A. Torres • D.A. Rodriguez • J. Gutierrez-Pajares • J.C. Tapia
FONDAP Center for Molecular Studies of the Cell (CEMC), Universidad de Chile,
Av. Independencia, 1027 Santiago, Chile
e-mail: aquest@med.uchile.cl

I. Mercier et al. (eds.), *Caveolins in Cancer Pathogenesis, Prevention and Therapy*,
Current Cancer Research, DOI 10.1007/978-1-4614-1001-0_2,
© Springer Science+Business Media, LLC 2012

Introduction

Caveolins are a family of membrane-associated scaffolding proteins implicated in a variety of functions in cells including vesicle trafficking, cholesterol transport, and regulation of signal transduction processes [2, 102, 112]. To date, three major isoforms have been described in mammals, namely caveolin-1, -2, and -3. Caveolin-1 and -2 are fairly generically expressed, while caveolin-3 presence is limited to muscle and glial cells [102, 116, 148]. All three isoforms are encoded by distinct genes [148]. Different variants have been described for caveolin-1 and -2. In the case of caveolin-2, function remains poorly defined [117, 140]. Since evidence available to date has predominantly linked changes in caveolin-1 to cancer, we will focus the discussion here on this isoform.

For caveolin-1, two variants referred to as caveolin-1α and -1β have been described that are generated by alternative initiation or splicing [72, 73, 124]. Caveolin-1β lacks the first 31 amino acids present in caveolin-1α, which also contains the amino acid tyrosine 14 that is phosphorylated by src family kinases [18, 77] in response to growth factors like insulin [71, 82, 97, 98] or EGF [82, 103] and by extracellular stimuli including, UV, oxidative stress, or hyperosmolarity [19, 89, 121, 141]. The latter observations have implicated caveolin-1 and phosphorylation on tyrosine 14 in cellular stress responses. Consistently with this notion, caveolin-1 knockout mice have a reduced lifespan and are less resistant to partial hepatectomy [35, 105].

Caveolin-1 and its phosphorylated form are also implicated in cell migration. A specific sequence (amino acids 46–55) is required for the localization to the rear of migrating cells [132, 133]. These events are important for polarized distribution of cell signaling elements and directional cell migration [8, 63, 104]. Although phosphorylation of caveolin-1 on tyrosine 14 has been shown to favor migration via a process involving recruitment of the adaptor protein Grb7 [82], the precise role of caveolin-1 in these events remains an issue of controversy due to technical problems associated with the definition of phospho-caveolin-1 localization in migrating cells [58].

Despite these issues, a large body of literature is available linking the expression of caveolin-1 not only to enhanced migration but also to metastasis of cancer cells. Likewise, caveolin-1 is implicated in development of the multidrug resistance (MDR) phenotype of aggressive cancer cells. All three characteristics of caveolin-1 mentioned, namely its participation in cellular stress responses and regeneration, migration and metastasis, as well as MDR tend to favor the interpretation that caveolin-1 represents a protein whose presence favors tumor development. Such evidence, however, has generated an intense discussion concerning the precise role of caveolin-1 in cancer, since also a large body of data is available in the literature suggesting that caveolin-1 functions as a tumor suppressor (see subsequent sections). A key objective of this chapter will be to highlight important aspects of this ongoing discussion and reconcile in a working model (see Fig. 2.3) these different and opposing functions of caveolin-1. In doing so, we will focus our attention mostly on studies dealing with the role of caveolin-1 in colorectal cancer. There, as will be eluded to in the next section, alterations in the so-called canonical Wnt signaling pathway are particularly important.

Canonical Wnt Signaling in Colorectal Cancer: The Role of β-Catenin

Colorectal cancer is one of the most common cancers and a leading cause of cancer death worldwide. By the age of 70, roughly 50% of the Western population develops polyps, some of which will progress to cancer. The lifetime risk of developing cancer in this population is estimated to be 5% [65]. Despite the fact that the incidence of this cancer has decreased in recent years as a result of the introduction of preventive measures, including the use of nonsteroidal anti-inflammatory drugs (NSAIDs) and changes in life-style and nutrition, the disease still remains a major threat. Every year, some 550,000 patients worldwide continue to succumb to the disease [49].

In molecular and genetic terms, colorectal cancer is likely to be one of the best-understood solid malignancies. The earliest detectable microscopic lesions are aberrant crypt foci, which progress over time to macroscopically detectable polyps. The transition to benign adenomas and then to malignant carcinomas is thought to be progressive. Our current molecular understanding of these events is strongly based on insights gained from hereditary forms of the disease that either involve mutations in the tumor suppressor protein *adenomatous polyposis coli* (APC, familial adenomatous polyposis (FAP) patients) or mismatch repair genes (hereditary non-polyposis colorectal cancer (HNPCC) patients). In the latter case, mutations in cancer causing genes, such as APC, are observed. Indeed, mutations in APC appear to represent a common event in a large majority of sporadic colon cancers, although the timing might vary considerably (reviewed in [114]). Despite such variations, the following sequence of events is invoked for the adenoma-carcinoma progression in colorectal cancer: First, colon tumors are thought to result from mutational activation of oncogenes (*K-ras, β-catenin*) and inactivation of tumor suppressor genes (APC and *P53 (TP53)*), whereby APC mutation is often an early event; second, the accumulation of several mutations is required to generate the disease; third mutations may occur in a preferential order. However, this is not required and it is the accumulation of specific mutations together with the associated survival-enhancing characteristics that are most relevant [51, 114]. Given the aforementioned importance of APC mutations in the genesis of colon cancer, it is perhaps not surprising that the canonical Wnt signaling pathway represents an important mechanism implicated in the etiology of both, inherited and sporadic colorectal cancers.

Wnt morphogens were originally described as factors involved in *Drosophila* development, and thereafter they became the focus of interest in other areas of research due to their implication in the development of human diseases like cancer. Two principle Wnt signaling pathways exist, referred to as the canonical and non-canonical pathways. For the non-canonical Wnt pathway, two variants have been described, the "Planar Cell Polarity" (PCP) pathway, which is important in the regulation of cytoskeletal changes associated with the development of the embryonic axis, and the "Calcium pathway," which regulates cell adhesion [144]. Alterations in all signaling pathways (canonical and non-canonical) have been associated with the development of cancer [6, 9, 12]. However, to date, caveolin-1 interactions predominantly with the canonical pathway have been reported. Thus, due to the focus of this book chapter, we will limit our discussion here to establishing connections between caveolin-1 and the canonical pathway, which still represents the best-characterized Wnt signaling pathway.

The canonical Wnt pathway is involved in the control of a large variety of processes, including cell proliferation, morphology, migration, and differentiation, all key events in the genesis and progression of cancer. A crucial molecular component in this pathway is the protein β-catenin [12, 109, 144]. A large number of studies in flies, frogs, and mammals have contributed to our current understanding of the importance of β-catenin turnover and localization for signaling via the canonical Wnt pathway (see Fig. 2.1). In non-stimulated cells, cytoplasmic free β-catenin is destabilized by the action of a multiprotein complex containing Axin/Conductin, glycogen synthase kinase 3β (GSK3β/Shaggy), and the tumor suppressor APC [12, 54, 56, 100, 109]. In this complex, Axin/Conductin acts as a scaffolding protein that binds APC, GSK3β, and β-catenin, thereby promoting the phosphorylation of APC and β-catenin, the latter being at specific serine and threonine residues located at the N-terminal end. Presence of the tumor suppressor p53 favors integration of Axin into this complex and hence phosphorylation of β-catenin [84].

Axin also associates with the protein kinase casein kinase 1 (CK1α), which phosphorylates β-catenin prior to GSK3β engagement and thereby promotes subsequent GSK3β-dependent phosphorylation, in a process referred to as hierarchical phosphorylation [54]. The importance of this sequence is substantiated by experiments showing that CK1α silencing causes abnormal embryogenesis due to excessive canonical Wnt signaling as the result of reduced β-catenin degradation [92]. Subsequent phosphorylation of β-catenin by GSK3β drives ubiquitination by the Skp1-Cul1-F-box-protein (SCF) complex, which contains the F-box protein βTrCP/Slimb that contacts the phosphorylated N-terminus of β-catenin and promotes its ubiquitination via an E3 ubiquitin ligase and subsequent proteasome-mediated degradation [70]. The exact role of APC in the complex remains unclear, although the C-terminal region of APC reportedly regulates β-catenin phosphorylation by GSK3β [120]. Also APC phosphorylation favors interactions with β-catenin that enhance its subsequent degradation by favoring nuclear export [50, 55, 56, 151].

Wnt-dependent activation of the pathway requires two transmembrane receptors, Frizzled and LRP5/6 (low-density lipoprotein receptor-related protein 5/6), which form a complex that triggers signaling to the cytoplasm and precludes β-catenin degradation [101]. The LRP5/6 co-receptor is sequentially phosphorylated at several PPPSP sites by CK1γ and GSK3β [155]. CK1γ association with LRP5/6 at the membrane is necessary and sufficient to transduce the signal in vertebrates [27]. Phosphorylation of LRP5/6 promotes recruitment of Axin and Disheveled (Dvl/Dsh), whereby the latter inhibits GSK3β in the complex and prevents phosphorylation of β-catenin, APC, and Axin. Nonphosphorylated β-catenin does not bind to βTrCP/Slimb and translocates to the nucleus, where it displaces Groucho, a repressor of T cell factor/lymphoid enhancer binding factor (Tcf/Lef) family of transcription factors. In doing so, the expression of many target genes involved in cell progression, viability, and resistance to apoptosis, such as *myc*, *cyclin D1*, *cox-2*, and *survivin*, is

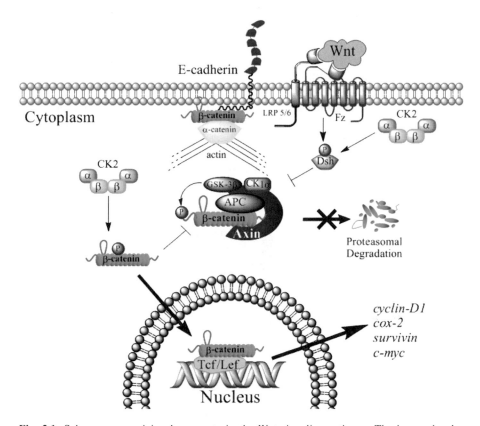

Fig. 2.1 Scheme summarizing key events in the Wnt signaling pathway. The key molecular component of this pathway is the protein β-catenin. In cells, β-catenin is found in three subcellular locations, the plasma membrane, the cytosol and the nucleus. At the plasma membrane, β-catenin is present in complexes with α-catenin and E-cadherin that are important for the regulation of cell–cell interactions and organization of the actin cytoskeleton. In the cytoplasm, β-catenin is part of a multiprotein complex containing Axin, adenomatous polyposis coli (APC), glycogen synthase kinase 3β (GSK3β), and casein kinase (CK1α). There, GSK3β phosphorylates β-catenin, which results in its ubiquitination and subsequent proteasome-mediated degradation. Wnt binding to Frizzled receptors (Fz) in association with co-receptors of the low-density lipoprotein receptor-related protein (LRP) family (LRP5/6) promotes Disheveled (Dvl) phosphorylation and thereby precludes β-catenin degradation. Additionally, CK2 can either phosphorylate and activate Dsh or directly phosphorylate β-catenin. Both canonical Wnt signaling and CK2-mediated events preclude β-catenin degradation and promote translocation to the nucleus. There, β-catenin acts as a transcriptional co-activator by associating with transcription factors of the T cell factor/lymphoid enhancer binding factor (Tcf/Lef) family and promotes the expression of a large number of genes, many of which are directly implicated in cancer, such as *cyclin-D1*, *cox-2*, *survivin* and *c-myc*. According to this model, both sequestration of β-catenin at the plasma membrane and degradation in the cytosol limit the amount of β-catenin available for translocation to the nucleus

enhanced [69, 75, 76, 96, 110, 134, 137, 138, 157]. More recently, β-catenin has also been suggested to function as a platform for the formation of chromatin-remodeling complexes [99].

Mutations in the N-terminus of β-catenin make it refractory to regulation by APC, decreasing phosphorylation of serine and threonine residues essential for degradation of β-catenin and thereby eliminating the phosphorylation-dependent interaction with β-transducin repeat containing protein (βTrCP). Mutations of the β-catenin N-terminus have been described in a number of human cancers, as well as in chemically- or genetically-induced animal tumor models. However, most tumors in colon cancer are associated with deletions at the C-terminal end of APC, while the frequency of mutations in β-catenin is surprisingly low [109].

In addition to the APC/axin complex that favors β-catenin degradation, another cytoplasmic complex exists that promotes the stabilization of β-catenin. This complex is thought to be activated by Wnt ligands and includes amongst others Dvl and the protein kinase CK2 as a central element [131]. CK2 is also suggested to participate as a critical component of the canonical Wnt pathway, since overexpression of this kinase mimics the dorsal axis development in *Xenopus* embryos probably by acting downstream of Gαq and Gα$_0$ and Dvl [29, 41]. By using immunoprecipitation, pull-down and in vitro activity assays, CK2 was shown to associate with and phosphorylate APC [131]. Notably, the same region of APC that is frequently deleted in colorectal cancers contains a sequence rich in basic residues that presumably inhibit the catalytic activity of CK2 [61]. CK2 inhibition by APC is thought to destabilize β-catenin, as well as Dvl and thereby block cell proliferation [131]. Protein kinase CK2 also interacts with and phosphorylates β-catenin, thereby increasing cytoplasmic stability [125, 130]. Consistent with these observations, CK2 overexpression promotes expression of the inhibitor of apoptosis protein (IAP) survivin, a known canonical Wnt target gene, while pharmacological CK2 inhibition decreases survivin expression [137]. Site-directed mutagenesis showed that phosphorylation of β-catenin by CK2 occurs mainly at threonine-393, where the proteins Axin and APC interact to promote its degradation [130]. Thus, CK2-phosphorylated β-catenin at residue 393 is thought to be protected from Axin and APC-dependent degradation, hence enhancing transcriptional activation [125].

Finally, ectopic expression of Wnt1 in the mammary gland cell line C57MG, as well as ectopic expression of CK2α in the same tissue from transgenic mice, revealed that this kinase associates with and phosphorylates Dvl, as well as stabilizes β-catenin. Thus, elevated CK2 levels are associated with increased proliferation and hyperplasia in vitro and in vivo [78, 79, 131]. Despite this evidence, several aspects concerning the mechanism by which CK2 positively regulates β-catenin are controversial. For instance, it remains unclear whether the regulatory effects require only the CK2α catalytic subunit- or the holoenzyme or whether all effects are associated exclusively with β-catenin phosphorylation. However, it is beyond the scope of this book chapter to discuss such aspects. The interested reader is referred to other studies which deal in more detail with these aspect [41, 125, 130, 131, 137, 142].

As outlined, the protein β-catenin is found at three principle intracellular locations: the membrane, the cytoplasm, and the nucleus. Association with protein complexes in the cytoplasm modulates the turnover of the protein, while presence in the nucleus is associated with transcription. An alternative mode to restrict translocation to the nucleus is by sequestration at the plasma membrane. There β-catenin is bound to cadherins (i.e., E-cadherin in epithelial cells) in a multiprotein complex that links the membrane to the actin cytoskeleton and is thought to stabilize β-catenin. E-cadherin is a transmembrane protein with an extracellular domain involved in the Ca^{2+}-dependent homophilic interactions between molecules on adjacent cells. The cytoplasmic domain binds the proteins α- and β-catenin (or plakoglobin), as well as p120-catenin in a multiprotein complex that connects to the actin cytoskeleton. In doing so, cadherins physically link neighboring cells to one another [44]. The complex also is involved in the formation and organization of functionally distinct cell junctions, such as tight and gap junctions, as well as desmosomes [48, 143]. All these macromolecular structures are mediators of signaling events between adjacent cells that contribute to phenomena important for epithelial homeostasis, such as contact inhibition [33]. Here, it is perhaps worth mentioning that although cadherin–catenin adhesive complexes are generally associated with β-catenin sequestration and stabilization, recent evidence suggests alternative, β-catenin phospho-destruction complexes exist at cell–cell contact sites that may also be relevant to tissue morphogenesis [95].

In summary, enhanced signaling via the canonical Wnt pathway due to genetic and epigenetic changes is considered a major factor contributing to the development of colon cancer. A central player in this pathway is β-catenin that, once in the nucleus, promotes transcription of cancer-related genes in association with the Tcf/Lef family of transcription factors. Of particular interest in the subsequent discussion will be *cox-2* and *survivin* as target genes. Limiting β-catenin access to the nucleus is hence crucial to controlling such activities. Essentially two different mechanisms have been described: one involving proteasome-mediated turnover and other by sequestration to the plasma membrane. Available evidence indicates that perturbations in any one of these two pathways favor development and progression of colon cancer. Hence, the following sections will center on the discussion of our current understanding of how caveolin-1 participates in this scenario.

Role of Caveolin-1 as Tumor Suppressor in Colorectal Cancer: Inhibition of β-Catenin-Tcf/Lef-Dependent Gene Expression

Over the previous 15 years, a large amount of data has become available associating the presence of caveolin-1 with tumor suppression. However, as will be discussed later on, the ability of caveolin-1 to act in this fashion depends on the cellular context. Thus, caveolin-1 can be considered a "conditional" tumor suppressor. In the following paragraphs, data favoring a role for caveolin-1 as a tumor suppressor will be briefly summarized before focusing the discussion particularly on linking this ability to control of Wnt signaling pathways.

Initially, oncogene-mediated transformation of NIH3T3 fibroblasts was correlated with reduced caveolin-1 mRNA and protein levels, and re-expression of the protein was sufficient to revert cell transformation [32, 74]. Likewise, selective loss of caveolin-1 expression using a siRNA approach was sufficient to transform NIH3T3 fibroblasts [40]. Furthermore, caveolin-1 expression is reduced in a number of human tumors, including lung, mammary, colon, and ovarian carcinomas, as well as ovarian sarcomas and osteosarcomas [10, 11, 17, 59, 83, 113, 145, 146]. Here too, re-expression of caveolin-1 frequently, but not always, reverts characteristics associated with the transformed phenotype [7, 67, 88, 136, 153, 154]. More recently, decreased caveolin-1 level has been reported for lymph node metastases from head and neck squamous cell carcinoma and restoration of caveolin-1 expression suppressed growth and metastasis [156].

Despite the fact that caveolin-1 depletion in mice knockout models does not affect overall viability, it is now clear that caveolin-1 absence increases lung and mammary hyperplasia, angiogenesis, as well as carcinogen-induced tumor formation in skin tissue [20, 30, 115, 147]. Also, increased mammary and intestinal stem cell proliferation is observed in caveolin-1 knockout mice and caveolin-1 was also recently shown to control neural stem cell proliferation [64]. Finally, stromal expression of caveolin-1 in breast cancer predicts outcome, recurrence, and survival, further highlighting its relevance as a potential therapeutic target [129, 150]. Indeed, caveolin-1 mutation on P132L, which was previously linked to breast cancer [53], was recently demonstrated to predict recurrence and metastasis in a mouse orthotopic model [13]. Taken together, these reports demonstrate that caveolin-1 displays traits consistent with a role as a tumor suppressor. This ability of caveolin-1 has often been linked to inhibition of signaling events associated with cell survival and proliferation. However, it is important to note that alternative mechanisms have also been proposed. For a more detailed discussion of literature related to the tumor suppressor hypothesis, the interested reader is referred to additional reviews [111, 149].

Initially, our entrance to the caveolin field came with the demonstration that caveolin-1 protein levels are reduced both in the mucosa and stroma of tumors from patients with colon cancer, as well as in colon adenocarcinoma cells and that caveolin-1 functions as a tumor suppressor in vivo upon re-expression in different colon adeno-carcinoma cells [10, 11]. Despite the ever-increasing abundance of signaling molecules available in the literature for regulation by caveolin-1 at the time, relatively few were linked to specific transcriptional events. Thus, as one approach, we set out to compare, by microarray analysis, colon cancer cell lines expressing or not caveolin-1. Rather intriguingly, those studies identified in an initial screen the IAP protein survivin as one of the most strongly down-regulated targets at the transcriptional level [138]. This protein is of tremendous interest, since it is abundantly expressed in a variety of human tumors including lung, colon, breast, prostate, pancreatic, and gastric carcinoma, but is essentially absent in most normal tissues. Importantly, survivin expression in cancer cells is linked to tumor survival. These characteristics define survivin as a tumor-specific antigen [1, 85, 118].

The difficulty, at the time, consisted in linking the expression of what was generally considered a plasma membrane bound scaffolding protein (caveolin-1) to specific transcriptional regulation. Suggestive hints in that respect came from two reports showing that caveolin-1 inhibits canonical Wnt signaling pathway by sequestering β-catenin to the plasma membrane and preventing the transcription of genes, such as *cyclin-D1* [39, 62]. Furthermore, the possibility that caveolin-1 might regulate *survivin* expression via the β-catenin pathway became all the more likely when *survivin* was identified as a β-catenin-Tcf/Lef target gene [69, 157]. Given the relevance of this pathway to the genesis of colon cancer, these results inspired the experiments that are summarized in a working model (see Fig. 2.2).

The following studies in a number of different cell lines, including human embryonic kidney cells (HEK293T), breast (ZR75), and colon (DLD-1) cancer cell lines, as well as mouse NIH3T3 fibroblasts confirmed the suspicion that caveolin-1 limited β-catenin-Tcf/Lef-dependent transcription of the *survivin* gene by a mechanism involving formation of a multiprotein complex and sequestration to the plasma membrane. Interestingly, limitations imposed on cells by the presence of caveolin-1 in terms of viability and proliferation were overcome by the re-expression of survivin [138]. These observations were subsequently confirmed in HT29 colon adenocarcinoma cells. Furthermore, the HT29 studies revealed that formation of caveolin-1/β-catenin multiprotein complexes at the cell surface required the presence of E-cadherin. In the absence of this protein, the ability of caveolin-1 to limit β-catenin-Tcf/Lef-dependent transcription of the *survivin* gene was lost. These findings were also shown to be valid in metastatic B16-F10 murine melanoma cells [139].

Given that many genes are regulated by the Wnt pathway, studies were initiated to identify other potentially interesting cancer-related genes. In this context, the analysis focused on Cyclooxygenase-2 (COX-2), a protein that is frequently up-regulated in cancer. Increased levels of COX-2 augment prostaglandin E_2 (PGE_2) production enhance β-catenin-Tcf/Lef-dependent transcription, cellular proliferation, and reduce apoptosis [21, 127, 128]. In human colorectal cancer cells, increased expression of COX-2 is also associated with cancer progression and phenotypic changes that promote metastasis. Interestingly, NSAIDs that specifically inhibit COX-2 activity have been shown to be quite effective in chemoprevention of FAP patients. Thus, COX-2 is of great interest as a target in cancer therapy [49].

As suspected, ectopic expression of caveolin-1 down-regulates also *cox-2* expression by suppression of β-catenin-Tcf/Lef-dependent transcription via sequestration of β-catenin to the plasma membrane. Interestingly, the presence of E-cadherin is also required here [119]. Several previous studies linked COX-2 and survivin expression, not only because they are both β-catenin-Tcf/Lef-dependent genes, but also because COX-2-dependent mechanisms involving PGE_2 are part of a positive feedback loop that potentiates signaling events linked to enhancing survivin levels (see Fig. 2.2). Regulation of survivin in this manner may also implicate post-transcriptional mechanisms [76]. Since loss of E-cadherin is frequently observed in human epithelial tumors [22], these studies suggested that the combined loss of caveolin-1 and E-cadherin in epithelial cells promotes increased expression of genes relevant to epithelial–mesenchymal transition, loss of cell–cell contacts, and cell transformation.

Perhaps even more importantly, they provide mechanistic insights to how caveolin-1-specific suppression of genes associated with its role as a tumor suppressor becomes "conditional," that is dependent on the cellular context [111, 139]. Interestingly, this ability of caveolin-1 is not only limited by the proteins present within cells expressing caveolin-1, but also by factors present in the cellular medium.

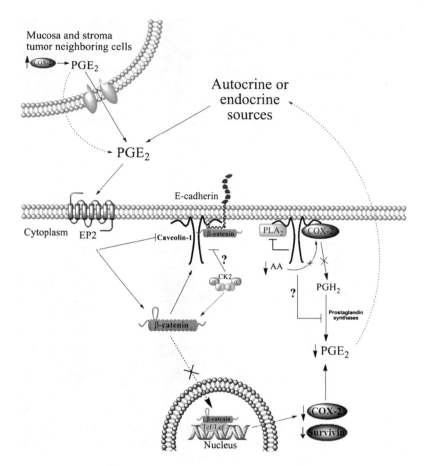

Fig. 2.2 Caveolin-1-mediated inhibition of the canonical Wnt and cyclooxygenase-2 (COX-2)/ prostaglandin E_2 (PGE$_2$) signaling pathways. Caveolin-1 presence promotes recruitment of β-catenin to the plasma membrane in association with E-cadherin, thereby decreasing β-catenin-Tcf/Lef-dependent transcriptional activity and the expression of genes like *cox-2* and *survivin*. Alternatively, caveolin-1 may inhibit phospholipase A_2 (PLA$_2$) and reduce the levels of arachidonic acid (AA), thereby limiting the ability of COX-2 to produce prostaglandin H_2 (PGH$_2$), or caveolin-1 may reduce the activity of prostaglandin synthases that convert PGH$_2$ to PGE$_2$. PGE$_2$ is depicted as acting in an autocrine or paracrine/endocrine fashion when derived from neighboring mucosa and/or stroma cells. Subsequently, PGE$_2$ can bind to receptors of the EP family (specifically depicted EP2) and thereby trigger signaling events that disrupt both the cytosolic complex that promotes β-catenin degradation and the caveolin-1-containing complex that sequesters β-catenin to the membrane. Both mechanisms enhance β-catenin-Tcf/Lef-dependent transcriptional activity and target gene expression. CK2 activity can also increase β-catenin-Tcf/Lef-dependent transcription. However, whether this ability is associated exclusively with regulation of the β-catenin degradation complex remains an open question. According to our model, reduced presence of caveolin-1 in tumor cells and/or the stroma compartment will generate an environment that facilitates COX-2 expression, PGE$_2$ production and β-catenin-Tcf/Lef-dependent transcription of cancer-related genes

In particular, caveolin-1 expression was shown to limit PGE_2 accumulation in the culture media of HEK293T, DLD-1, and HT29 cells. Moreover, supplementation of media with PGE_2 disrupted caveolin-1-complexes responsible for sequestration of β-catenin to the plasma membrane [119].

Although our recent findings suggested that caveolin-1 presence decreased COX-2 expression and PGE_2 levels via a transcriptional mechanism [119], other possible scenarios by which caveolin-1 may decrease PGE_2 levels must be considered, given that PGE_2 is produced by the concerted action of several enzymes. Initially, arachidonic acid (AA) is generated by phospholipase A_2 (PLA_2) and converted to prostaglandin H_2 (PGH_2) by COX-2. PGH_2 is then specifically converted to PGE_2 by the prostaglandin synthase E_2 [106]. Thus, caveolin-1 may also interfere with any of these intermediate steps. Interestingly, in this context, caveolin-1 co-localizes both with PLA_2 [47] and COX-2 [91, 108] in caveolae [47, 108]. Moreover, caveolin-1 co-fractionates and co-immunoprecipitates with both proteins [43, 91]. Importantly, caveolin-1 inhibits the enzymatic activity of PLA_2 and decreases AA production via an interaction with the "caveolin-1 scaffolding domain (CSD)" [43], although the enzymatic activity of COX-2 appears not to be affected [91]. Thus, in addition to the aforementioned process of transcriptional regulation, one may envisage a scenario in which association of caveolin-1 with PLA_2 and/or COX-2, possibly in a common complex, will reduce PGH_2 availability and PGE_2 production. Hence, our model (Fig. 2.2) depicts both these mechanisms as possibilities by which caveolin-1 may inhibit PGE_2 production.

Additionally, PGE_2 is exported through the plasma membrane, either by passive diffusion or by active transport, for example via the multidrug resistant protein 4 (MDR-4) [106], which is overexpressed in some colon cancer cell lines [60]. Thus, we cannot rule out the possibility that caveolin-1 may also modulate PGE_2 transport from the cytosol to the extracellular space (see Fig. 2.2).

In summary, loss of caveolin-1 is associated, at least early on, with the development of some tumors. A majority of the data available suggests that this is the result of transcriptional silencing of caveolin-1 gene by epigenetic mechanisms (reviewed in [111]). The findings related to E-cadherin and PGE_2 highlight the existence of alternative modes of restricting caveolin-1 function that do not rely on gene silencing. Instead, the ability of caveolin-1 to function as a tumor suppressor appears limited by both intracellular and environmental factors [111, 119]. The latter observations suggest that inflammatory processes and events occurring in adjacent stroma cells are likely to be highly relevant to the role caveolin-1 plays in epithelial cells, both in early and later stages of tumor development. In this context, it is important to note that caveolin-1 protein levels are reduced in both the mucosa and stroma from tumors when compared with the same samples from normal colon tissue [11]. In view of these observations, it is intriguing to speculate that alterations in caveolin-1, not only in the epithelial compartment, are likely to be relevant to the genesis of colon and other cancers. Furthermore, once liberated from complexes, for instance with E-cadherin, caveolin-1 would be free to engage in other activities not necessarily related to tumor suppression (see following sections).

Caveolin-1 Expression in Colon Cancer: Tissue Analysis

The human intestine is divided anatomically into two segments, the small and the large intestine, whereby the first is considerably longer (6–7 m in an adult) than the second (roughly 1.5 m). Both segments are composed of several layers, including the mucosa (glandular epithelium and muscularis mucosa), submucosa, muscularis externa (inner circular and outer longitudinal), and lastly the serosa. As might be expected based on the presence of a considerable variety of cells in this tissue, including epithelial and muscle cells (see section "Introduction"), all three isoforms (caveolin-1, -2, and -3) have been detected in both intestinal segments [90]. Results from the literature suggest that caveolin-1 and -2 are expressed in epithelial cells of the small intestine and colon (Table 2.1).

Most available studies have focused on the analysis of caveolin-1 in the human colon; however, data are controversial. On the one hand, caveolin-1 is reportedly present in normal colon mucosa, as well as stroma and expression is reduced in tumors of different stages [11]. On the other hand, data arguing that caveolin-1 levels are elevated in colon tumor samples has also been provided [37, 107]. Specifically, caveolin-1 expression was increased in samples of adenocarcinomas, but not adenomas and normal mucosa [37]. Studies in rodents investigating the role of caveolin-1 in colon carcinogenesis are generally scarce. In one such study, caveolin-1, but not caveolin-2, expression increased in a rat model of adenocarcinoma induced by azoxymethane [107]. To the contrary, however, another study using caveolin-1 knock-out mice points to a role for caveolin-1 in controlling proliferation of intestinal crypt stem cells [86]. Clearly more experiments are required to clarify these discrepancies concerning caveolin-1 expression and function in humans and rodent models.

A review of the literature summarizing data available concerning caveolin expression in human, mouse, and rat intestine is shown in Table 2.1. In the majority of these studies, caveolin-1 mRNA and protein were detected in the mucosa of the intestine, specifically in epithelial cells [4, 5, 11, 36, 94]. Studies in tumors also offer controversial data, indicating that caveolin-1 may decrease in mucosa and stromal cells [11] or increase in epithelial cells [37] and in distant metastases [66].

Caveolin-1 Expression in Colon Cancer: Human Colon Cancer Cell Lines

The aforementioned controversy concerning caveolin-1 expression is further highlighted by the situation in cell lines (see Table 2.2). For a number of colon adenocarcinoma cells (HT29, DLD-1, Lovo, Col12, SW480, SW620), low caveolin-1 expression levels have been reported [11, 15, 107], while for others (T84, HCT116) caveolin-1 levels are readily detectable [5, 23, 36, 107]. A number of possible

Table 2.1 Expression of caveolin-1 and caveolin-2 in intestinal tissues

Pathological status	Species	Segment	Cell type or tissue analyzed	Caveolin isoform	Detection method	References
Normal	H	SI	EpiC	Cav-1	WB, IHC, RT-PCR	[5]
Normal	H	SI	EpiC	Cav-2	RT-PCR	[5]
Normal	H	SI, CR	Whole tissue	Cav-1	NB	[11]
Normal	H	SI		Cav-1	WB, RT-PCR	[36]
Normal	H	CR	SMC, EnC	Cav-1	IHC	[4]
Normal	H	CR	N.d.	Cav-2	IHC	[4]
Normal	H	CR	Mucosa/Stroma	Cav-1	WB	[11]
Normal	H	CR	EpiC	↓ Cav-1	IHC	[37]
Normal	H	CR	EnC	Cav-1	IHC	[37]
Normal	M	CR	EpiC	Cav-1	WB	[94]
Inflammation	H	CR	SMC, EnC	Cav-1	IHC	[4]
Inflammation	H	CR	EpiC	↑ Cav-2	IHC	[4]
Adenoma	H	CR	EpiC	↓ Cav-1	IHC	[37]
Carcinoma	H	CR	Mucosa	↓ Cav-1	WB	[11]
		CR	Stroma	↓ Cav-1	WB	[11]
Carcinoma	H	CR	Glands	↑ Cav-1	IHC	[37]
Carcinoma	H	CR		↑ Cav-1	IHC	[66]
Carcinoma	H	CR	Tumor	↑ Cav-1	RT-PCR	[68]
Experimental carcinoma	R	CR	Mucosa	↑ Cav-1	WB, RT-PCR	[107]
Distant metastasis	H	CR	Mucosa	↑ Cav-1	IHC	[66]

Species: *H* human; *M* mouse; *R* rat

Segment: *SI* small intestine; *CR* colorectum

Cell type: *SMC* smooth muscle cell; *EnC* endothelial cell; *EpiC* epithelial cell

Detection method: *WB* Western blotting; *IHC* immunohistochemistry; *RT-PCR* reverse transcription-polymerase chain reaction; *NB* Northern blot

N.d. Analyzed but not detected

Table 2.2 Expression of caveolin-1 and caveolin-2 in human colorectal carcinoma cell lines

Cell line	Source[a]	Caveolin isoform	Detection method	References
T84	Colorectal carcinoma derived from lung	Cav-1	WB/RT-PCR	[5]
		Cav-2	RT-PCR	[5]
Caco-2	Colorectal adenocarcinoma	↓ Cav-1	WB/NB	[11, 15]
		↓ Cav-1	WB	[107]
		Cav-1	WB, IHC, RT-PCR	[36]
		↓ Cav-2	WB	[15]
Caco-2E	Colorectal adenocarcinoma	Cav-1	WB/RT-PCR	[5]
		Cav-2	RT-PCR	[5]
HCT116	Colorectal adenocarcinoma	Cav-1	WB	[23]
		Cav-1	WB	[57]
		Cav-1	WB, RT-PCR	[107]
HT29	Colorectal adenocarcinoma	↓ Cav-1	WB/NB	[11, 15, 16]
		Cav-1	WB, RT-PCR	[107]
HT29-MDR	Colorectal adenocarcinoma	↑ Cav-1	WB	[80]
		↑ Cav-2	WB	[80]
SW480	Colorectal adenocarcinoma (Dukes' type B)	↓ Cav-1	WB/NB	[11, 25]
SW620	Colorectal adenocarcinoma derived from lymph node (Dukes' type C)	↓ Cav-1	WB/NB	[11]
Col12		↓ Cav-1	WB/NB	[11]
DLD-1	Colorectal adenocarcinoma (Dukes' type C)	↓ Cav-1	WB/NB	[11]

[a]Data obtained from ATCC web site (http://www.atcc.org)
Tumor stage in brackets

explanations may help explain these often contradictory observations. For instance, Caco-2 cells have been observed both to express or not caveolin-1 (Table 2.2). These variations may be linked to cell passaging, since differences in caveolin-1 expression have been reported for Caco-2 with low (Caco-2E) and high passage numbers (Caco-2L) [93]. Also, augmented caveolin-1 levels in colon cancer cell lines have been associated with MDR and elevated metastatic potential. For instance, HT29-MDR cells obtained by selecting HT29 cells for growth in increasing concentrations of colchicine [14] or HT29-5M21 and M12 cells obtained from HT29 cells by selection in the presence of methotrexate [11] all have elevated caveolin-1 levels with respect to HT29 cells. Alternatively, cells with elevated metastatic potential, such as Lovo E2 and C5 as well as HT29(US), express higher caveolin-1 levels than the reference lines, Lovo and HT29(ATCC), respectively [11, 139]. Finally, caveolin-1 expression levels may vary quite dramatically upon exposure of colon and other cancer cells to different stress situations, including the addition of hydrogen peroxide (Gutierrez-Pajares and Quest, unpublished data).

Indeed, similar variations in caveolin-1 expression linked to MDR and metastasis have also been observed in other cancer cell lines. Likewise, a significant amount of data is available in the literature associating elevated caveolin-1 levels in prostate, breast, and other cancers with angiogenesis, aggressive cancer recurrence, enhanced metastasis and generally reduced patient survival (reviewed in [111]). More recently, caveolin-1 was found to represent an independent predictor of decreased survival and higher metastatic potential, not only in colon, but also in breast cancer [66]. Moreover, gene expression profiling identified caveolin-1, together with PKCα and Enolase 2 as the main targets up-regulated in HT29 cells resistant to methotrexate, while E-cadherin was repressed in resistant cells [126]. This result is remarkably similar to the aforementioned situation in HT29 cells, where HT29(US) with elevated metastatic potential, unlike the original HT29(ATCC) cells, essentially lack E-cadherin, but have modestly increased (roughly fivefold) caveolin-1 levels [139]. Interestingly, siRNA-mediated targeting of caveolin-1 decreased viability of resistant cells in the presence of methotrexate and reconstitution of E-cadherin in addition to caveolin-1 depletion further sensitized these cells to the chemotherapeutic drugs [126].

In summary, these observations may be taken to indicate that caveolin-1 levels can fluctuate considerably depending on the circumstances. Consistent with this possibility, a large number of mechanisms have been described that may either promote or suppress caveolin-1 expression in both non-transformed and cancer cell lines (reviewed in [111]).

The Ambiguous Role of Caveolin-1 in Cancer

Despite the abundance of evidence summarized previously indicating that caveolin-1 functions as a tumor suppressor, there is also evidence suggesting a radically different, even opposite role for caveolin-1. This potentially conflicting interpretation of data in the literature already became apparent from the summary provided concerning the expression of caveolin-1 in colon tissue and cancer cell lines (see previous section). Furthermore, caveolin-1 is known to promote tumor formation and its presence is correlated with poor prognosis and survival in prostate cancer. Indeed, the expression of caveolin-1 reportedly increases in primary tumors from prostate [154] and certain leukemia-derived cell lines [52]. Also, in prostate cancer cells, caveolin-1 presence increases tumor growth and the incidence of metastasis [7, 67, 88, 136]. Increased caveolin-1 expression in tumor samples is not restricted to cases, like the prostate, where normal tissues have low relative caveolin-1 levels, since increased expression was also reported in tumor models where initial caveolin-1 loss is observed, such as colon [11] and breast cancer [38, 42, 123]. In most of these cases, the available data argue for a strong positive correlation between expression of caveolin-1, metastasis, and MDR [42, 80, 81]. Moreover, studies in samples derived from esophageal squamous cell carcinoma [3], small cell lung carcinomas [59], colon cancer cells with high metastatic potential ([11], see below) and gastric cancer [16], revealed that caveolin-1 expression correlates with poor patient prognosis. Furthermore, caveolin-1 is also overexpressed in nasopharyngeal carcinoma and protein levels correlate there with poor prognosis, enhanced tumor cell migration, and metastasis [31]. Finally, caveolin-1 was recently associated with tumor promotion in a panel of melanoma cell lines, since increased expression correlated with enhanced proliferation, cell migration, and tumorigenicity [34].

A variety of mechanisms have been proposed to explain how caveolin-1 may promote tumorigenesis. As so often, these depend on the tumor model under study. For example, in prostate cancer cells, increased caveolin-1 levels were found to favor growth factor release and regulation by a positive feedback loop that enhances tumor cell invasiveness [87] and VEGF-associated angiogenic signaling [135]. In breast cancer cells, caveolin-1 was recently shown to associate with type 1 matrix metalloproteinase, both promoting invadopodia formation and matrix degradation, thereby providing a mechanism explaining increased invasiveness [152]. Indeed, caveolin-1 increased hepatocellular carcinoma cell motility and invasiveness was associated with augmented metalloproteinase expression and secretion together with down-regulation of E-cadherin [26]. Successful tumor cell migration requires proper cell polarization, directionality, and the ability to invade new surrounding matrices. Importantly, caveolin-1 is known to promote cell polarization and directional migration in different experimental settings [8, 104]. Indeed, in transmigrating endothelial cells, caveolin-1 was shown to interact with intermediate filaments [122]. In support of this, a body of evidence involves caveolin-1 in regulating the small GTPases Rho and Rac, which are required for actin dynamics, cell polarization, and directional migration [28, 45, 46].

The role of caveolin-1 in tumorigenesis has not only focused on mechanisms of migration and invasiveness. It was recently suggested that in human lung carcinoma cells, caveolin-1 undergoes proteasome-dependent degradation during anoikis, and resistance induced by nitric oxide involves decreased caveolin-1 ubiquitination and impairment of apoptotic responses [24].

Taken together, the data summarized in this section collectively support the view that caveolin-1 expression is linked to the acquisition of traits associated with malignant cell behavior, including MDR and metastasis, as well as poor patient prognosis in the clinic (see Fig. 2.3).

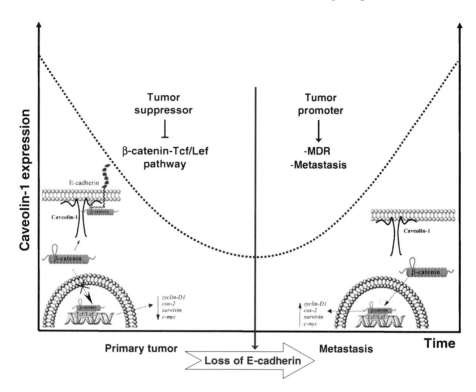

Fig. 2.3 Dual role of caveolin-1 in tumorigenesis. In colon cancer, loss of caveolin-1 is depicted as correlating initially with enhanced β-catenin-dependent transcription and the acquisition of traits associated with tumor development, including increased proliferation and decreased apoptosis. Re-introduction of caveolin-1 into tumor cells that still express E-cadherin (early stages of tumor development) leads to the repression of β-catenin-Tcf/Lef-dependent transcription of genes, such as *cyclin D1, cox-2, survivin* and *c-myc*. However, during tumor progression multiple changes occur at the molecular level (i.e., genome instability, genetic mutations and/or epigenetic alterations). One such possibility is the loss of E-cadherin. In this now "permissive" cellular environment, caveolin-1 can no longer repress pathways associated with its role as a tumor suppressor, including the canonical Wnt signaling pathway. Instead, traits of the molecule prevail that favor the development of multi-drug resistance (MDR) and metastasis. This view is consistent with data in the literature associating caveolin-1 expression at later stages of tumor development with higher metastatic potential, MDR and poor patient survival. Finally, our model reinforces the view that caveolin-1 is a "conditional" tumor suppressor and that its ability to promote or suppress tumor development depend both on the cellular context and environmental conditions

The Caveolin-1 Conundrum: Summary and Outlook

The data summarized here reinforce the notion that caveolin-1 plays a dual role in cancer (reviewed in [111, 112]). The ambiguity of caveolin-1 function is perhaps best reconciled by the view portrayed for colon cancer in Fig. 2.3. An initial loss of caveolin-1 is depicted as being followed by re-expression at later stages. Early on the cellular environment is such that if caveolin-1 is re-expressed, it develops traits consistent with a role as a tumor suppressor. In our model, regulation of the Wnt signaling pathway is depicted as one possibility. Surely, many more are likely to exist. During tumor progression, the cellular context changes, since expression of a large number of proteins is altered. One such possibility highlighted here is the loss of E-cadherin. Bearing in mind the effects of the PGE_2 that were discussed, it is important to note that not only "intracellular" but also "extracellular" changes need to be considered. The latter may represent the consequence of events occurring within the tumor cell itself, the stroma compartment or both. Later, if caveolin-1 expression is triggered by events that remain as yet poorly defined, the protein will no longer encounter a cellular environment conducive to its role as a tumor suppressor, indicated here as the loss of its ability to suppress β-catenin-dependent transcription. Instead, other characteristics of the protein prevail, favoring the acquisition of characteristics associated with malignant cell behavior.

Although complex, the emerging picture is beginning to reconcile a large amount of data that at first sight appear contradictory. In doing so, the traditional view of cancer as a disease dominated by the interplay between oncogenes and tumor suppressors is blurring. Clearly, this image in black and white needs refining. Hence, learning more about such details by investigating caveolin-1 is likely to bring a great deal of insight to cancer biology per se. Two immediate needs in caveolin-1 research have become apparent. First, we need to improve our knowledge of what "environmental" and "cellular" components determine whether caveolin-1 functions one way or another. Second, a specific understanding of the elements within the protein that are required in vivo for the molecule to act as a tumor suppressor or promote opposing characteristics in a tumor cell is essential. With these insights at hand, we can expect to initiate the design and use of successful caveolin-1-based strategies in the treatment of cancer.

Acknowledgments The work was supported by the FONDAP grant #15010006, ICGEB grant CRP/CH108-03 (to A.F.G.Q), FONDECYT grants: #1090071 (to A.F.G.Q), #1095234 and #11070116 (to J.C.T.), #3100033 (to D.R.G).

References

1. Altieri DC (2003) Validating survivin as a cancer therapeutic target. Nat Rev Cancer 3:46–54
2. Anderson RG (1998) The caveolae membrane system. Annu Rev Biochem 67:199–225
3. Ando T, Ishiguro H, Kimura M et al (2007) The overexpression of caveolin-1 and caveolin-2 correlates with a poor prognosis and tumor progression in esophageal squamous cell carcinoma. Oncol Rep 18:601–609
4. Andoh A, Saotome T, Sato H et al (2001) Epithelial expression of caveolin-2, but not caveolin-1, is enhanced in the inflamed mucosa of patients with ulcerative colitis. Inflamm Bowel Dis 7:210–214
5. Badizadegan K, Dickinson BL, Wheeler HE et al (2000) Heterogeneity of detergent-insoluble membranes from human intestine containing caveolin-1 and ganglioside G(M1). Am J Physiol Gastrointest Liver Physiol 278:G895–G904
6. Barker N, Clevers H (2000) Catenins, Wnt signaling and cancer. Bioessays 22:961–965

7. Bartz R, Zhou J, Hsieh JT et al (2008) Caveolin-1 secreting LNCaP cells induce tumor growth of caveolin-1 negative LNCaP cells in vivo. Int J Cancer 122:520–525
8. Beardsley A, Fang K, Mertz H et al (2005) Loss of caveolin-1 polarity impedes endothelial cell polarization and directional movement. J Biol Chem 280:3541–3547
9. Behrens J (2000) Control of beta-catenin signaling in tumor development. Ann N Y Acad Sci 910:21–33; discussion 33–5
10. Bender F, Montoya M, Monardes V et al (2002) Caveolae and caveolae-like membrane domains in cellular signaling and disease: identification of downstream targets for the tumor suppressor protein caveolin-1. Biol Res 35:151–167
11. Bender FC, Reymond MA, Bron C et al (2000) Caveolin-1 levels are down-regulated in human colon tumors, and ectopic expression of caveolin-1 in colon carcinoma cell lines reduces cell tumorigenicity. Cancer Res 60:5870–5878
12. Bienz M, Clevers H (2000) Linking colorectal cancer to Wnt signaling. Cell 103:311–320
13. Bonuccelli G, Casimiro MC, Sotgia F et al (2009) Caveolin-1 (P132L), a common breast cancer mutation, confers mammary cell invasiveness and defines a novel stem cell/metastasis-associated gene signature. Am J Pathol 174:1650–1662
14. Breuer W, Slotki IN, Ausiello DA et al (1993) Induction of multidrug resistance downregulates the expression of CFTR in colon epithelial cells. Am J Physiol 265:C1711–C1715
15. Breuza L, Corby S, Arsanto JP et al (2002) The scaffolding domain of caveolin 2 is responsible for its Golgi localization in Caco-2 cells. J Cell Sci 115:4457–4467
16. Burgermeister E, Tencer L, Liscovitch M (2003) Peroxisome proliferator-activated receptor-gamma upregulates caveolin-1 and caveolin-2 expression in human carcinoma cells. Oncogene 22:3888–3900
17. Cantiani L, Manara MC, Zucchini C et al (2007) Caveolin-1 reduces osteosarcoma metastases by inhibiting c-Src activity and met signaling. Cancer Res 67:7675–7685
18. Cao H, Courchesne WE, Mastick CC (2002) A phosphotyrosine-dependent protein interaction screen reveals a role for phosphorylation of caveolin-1 on tyrosine 14: recruitment of C-terminal Src kinase. J Biol Chem 277:8771–8774
19. Cao H, Sanguinetti AR, Mastick CC (2004) Oxidative stress activates both Src-kinases and their negative regulator Csk and induces phosphorylation of two targeting proteins for Csk: caveolin-1 and paxillin. Exp Cell Res 294:159–171
20. Capozza F, Williams TM, Schubert W et al (2003) Absence of caveolin-1 sensitizes mouse skin to carcinogen-induced epidermal hyperplasia and tumor formation. Am J Pathol 162:2029–2039
21. Castellone MD, Teramoto H, Williams BO et al (2005) Prostaglandin E2 promotes colon cancer cell growth through a Gs-axin-beta-catenin signaling axis. Science 310:1504–1510
22. Cavallaro U, Christofori G (2004) Cell adhesion and signalling by cadherins and Ig-CAMs in cancer. Nat Rev Cancer 4:118–132
23. Cavallo-Medved D, Mai J, Dosescu J et al (2005) Caveolin-1 mediates the expression and localization of cathepsin B, pro-urokinase plasminogen activator and their cell-surface receptors in human colorectal carcinoma cells. J Cell Sci 118:1493–1503
24. Chanvorachote P, Nimmannit U, Lu Y et al (2009) Nitric oxide regulates lung carcinoma cell anoikis through inhibition of ubiquitin-proteasomal degradation of caveolin-1. J Biol Chem 284:28476–28484
25. Chintharlapalli S, Papineni S, Safe S (2006) 1,1-Bis(3′-indolyl)-1-(p-substituted phenyl) methanes inhibit colon cancer cell and tumor growth through PPARgamma-dependent and PPARgamma-independent pathways. Mol Cancer Ther 5:1362–1370
26. Cokakli M, Erdal E, Nart D et al (2009) Differential expression of caveolin-1 in hepatocellular carcinoma: correlation with differentiation state, motility and invasion. BMC Cancer 9:65
27. Davidson G, Wu W, Shen J et al (2005) Casein kinase 1 gamma couples Wnt receptor activation to cytoplasmic signal transduction. Nature 438:867–872
28. del Pozo MA, Balasubramanian N, Alderson NB et al (2005) Phospho-caveolin-1 mediates integrin-regulated membrane domain internalization. Nat Cell Biol 7:901–908

29. Dominguez I, Mizuno J, Wu H et al (2004) Protein kinase CK2 is required for dorsal axis formation in *Xenopus* embryos. Dev Biol 274:110–124
30. Drab M, Verkade P, Elger M et al (2001) Loss of caveolae, vascular dysfunction, and pulmonary defects in caveolin-1 gene-disrupted mice. Science 293:2449–2452
31. Du ZM, Hu CF, Shao Q et al (2009) Upregulation of caveolin-1 and CD147 expression in nasopharyngeal carcinoma enhanced tumor cell migration and correlated with poor prognosis of the patients. Int J Cancer 125:1832–1841
32. Engelman JA, Wykoff CC, Yasuhara S et al (1997) Recombinant expression of caveolin-1 in oncogenically transformed cells abrogates anchorage-independent growth. J Biol Chem 272:16374–16381
33. Fagotto F, Gumbiner BM (1996) Cell contact-dependent signaling. Dev Biol 180:445–454
34. Felicetti F, Parolini I, Bottero L et al (2009) Caveolin-1 tumor-promoting role in human melanoma. Int J Cancer 125:1514–1522
35. Fernandez MA, Albor C, Ingelmo-Torres M et al (2006) Caveolin-1 is essential for liver regeneration. Science 313:1628–1632
36. Field FJ, Born E, Murthy S et al (1998) Caveolin is present in intestinal cells: role in cholesterol trafficking? J Lipid Res 39:1938–1950
37. Fine SW, Lisanti MP, Galbiati F et al (2001) Elevated expression of caveolin-1 in adenocarcinoma of the colon. Am J Clin Pathol 115:719–724
38. Fiucci G, Ravid D, Reich R et al (2002) Caveolin-1 inhibits anchorage-independent growth, anoikis and invasiveness in MCF-7 human breast cancer cells. Oncogene 21:2365–2375
39. Galbiati F, Volonte D, Brown AM et al (2000) Caveolin-1 expression inhibits Wnt/beta-catenin/Lef-1 signaling by recruiting beta-catenin to caveolae membrane domains. J Biol Chem 275:23368–23377
40. Galbiati F, Volonte D, Engelman JA et al (1998) Targeted downregulation of caveolin-1 is sufficient to drive cell transformation and hyperactivate the p42/44 MAP kinase cascade. EMBO J 17:6633–6648
41. Gao Y, Wang HY (2006) Casein kinase 2 is activated and essential for wnt/beta-catenin signaling. J Biol Chem 281(27):18394–18400
42. Garcia S, Dales JP, Charafe-Jauffret E et al (2007) Poor prognosis in breast carcinomas correlates with increased expression of targetable CD146 and c-Met and with proteomic basal-like phenotype. Hum Pathol 38:830–841
43. Gaudreault SB, Chabot C, Gratton JP et al (2004) The caveolin scaffolding domain modifies 2-amino-3-hydroxy-5-methyl-4-isoxazole propionate receptor binding properties by inhibiting phospholipase A2 activity. J Biol Chem 279:356–362
44. Gottardi CJ, Wong E, Gumbiner BM (2001) E-cadherin suppresses cellular transformation by inhibiting beta-catenin signaling in an adhesion-independent manner. J Cell Biol 153:1049–1060
45. Grande-Garcia A, del Pozo MA (2008) Caveolin-1 in cell polarization and directional migration. Eur J Cell Biol 87:641–647
46. Grande-Garcia A, Echarri A, de Rooij J et al (2007) Caveolin-1 regulates cell polarization and directional migration through Src kinase and Rho GTPases. J Cell Biol 177:683–694
47. Graziani A, Bricko V, Carmignani M et al (2004) Cholesterol- and caveolin-rich membrane domains are essential for phospholipase A2-dependent EDHF formation. Cardiovasc Res 64:234–242
48. Gumbiner B (1988) Cadherins: a family of Ca2+−dependent adhesion molecules. Trends Biochem Sci 13:75–76
49. Gupta RA, Dubois RN (2001) Colorectal cancer prevention and treatment by inhibition of cyclooxygenase-2. Nat Rev Cancer 1:11–21
50. Ha NC, Tonozuka T, Stamos JL et al (2004) Mechanism of phosphorylation-dependent binding of APC to beta-catenin and its role in beta-catenin degradation. Mol Cell 15:511–521
51. Hanahan D, Weinberg RA (2000) The hallmarks of cancer. Cell 100:57–70
52. Hatanaka M, Maeda T, Ikemoto T et al (1998) Expression of caveolin-1 in human T cell leukemia cell lines. Biochem Biophys Res Commun 253:382–387
53. Hayashi K, Matsuda S, Machida K et al (2001) Invasion activating caveolin-1 mutation in human scirrhous breast cancers. Cancer Res 61:2361–2364

54. Heeg-Truesdell E, LaBonne C (2006) Wnt signaling: a shaggy dogma tale. Curr Biol 16:R62–R64
55. Henderson BR (2000) Nuclear-cytoplasmic shuttling of APC regulates beta-catenin subcellular localization and turnover. Nat Cell Biol 2:653–660
56. Henderson BR, Fagotto F (2002) The ins and outs of APC and beta-catenin nuclear transport. EMBO Rep 3:834–839
57. Henkhaus RS, Roy UK, Cavallo-Medved D et al (2008) Caveolin-1-mediated expression and secretion of kallikrein 6 in colon cancer cells. Neoplasia 10:140–148
58. Hill MM, Scherbakov N, Schiefermeier N et al (2007) Reassessing the role of phosphocaveolin-1 in cell adhesion and migration. Traffic 8:1695–1705
59. Ho CC, Huang PH, Huang HY et al (2002) Up-regulated caveolin-1 accentuates the metastasis capability of lung adenocarcinoma by inducing filopodia formation. Am J Pathol 161:1647–1656
60. Holla VR, Backlund MG, Yang P et al (2008) Regulation of prostaglandin transporters in colorectal neoplasia. Cancer Prev Res (Phila) 1:93–99
61. Homma MK, Li D, Krebs EG et al (2002) Association and regulation of casein kinase 2 activity by adenomatous polyposis coli protein. Proc Natl Acad Sci USA 99:5959–5964
62. Hulit J, Bash T, Fu M et al (2000) The cyclin D1 gene is transcriptionally repressed by caveolin-1. J Biol Chem 275:21203–21209
63. Isshiki M, Ando J, Yamamoto K et al (2002) Sites of Ca(2+) wave initiation move with caveolae to the trailing edge of migrating cells. J Cell Sci 115:475–484
64. Jasmin JF, Yang M, Iacovitti L et al (2009) Genetic ablation of caveolin-1 increases neural stem cell proliferation in the subventricular zone (SVZ) of the adult mouse brain. Cell Cycle 8:3978–3983
65. Jemal A, Thomas A, Murray T et al (2002) Cancer statistics, 2002. CA Cancer J Clin 52:23–47
66. Joshi B, Strugnell SS, Goetz JG et al (2008) Phosphorylated caveolin-1 regulates Rho/ROCK-dependent focal adhesion dynamics and tumor cell migration and invasion. Cancer Res 68:8210–8220
67. Karam JA, Lotan Y, Roehrborn CG et al (2007) Caveolin-1 overexpression is associated with aggressive prostate cancer recurrence. Prostate 67:614–622
68. Kim HA, Kim KH, Lee RA (2006) Expression of caveolin-1 is correlated with Akt-1 in colorectal cancer tissues. Exp Mol Pathol 80:165–170
69. Kim PJ, Plescia J, Clevers H et al (2003) Survivin and molecular pathogenesis of colorectal cancer. Lancet 362:205–209
70. Kimelman D, Xu W (2006) Beta-catenin destruction complex: insights and questions from a structural perspective. Oncogene 25:7482–7491
71. Kimura A, Mora S, Shigematsu S et al (2002) The insulin receptor catalyzes the tyrosine phosphorylation of caveolin-1. J Biol Chem 277:30153–30158
72. Kogo H, Aiba T, Fujimoto T (2004) Cell type-specific occurrence of caveolin-1alpha and -1beta in the lung caused by expression of distinct mRNAs. J Biol Chem 279:25574–25581
73. Kogo H, Fujimoto T (2000) Caveolin-1 isoforms are encoded by distinct mRNAs. Identification Of mouse caveolin-1 mRNA variants caused by alternative transcription initiation and splicing. FEBS Lett 465:119–123
74. Koleske AJ, Baltimore D, Lisanti MP (1995) Reduction of caveolin and caveolae in oncogenically transformed cells. Proc Natl Acad Sci USA 92:1381–1385
75. Krysan K, Dalwadi H, Sharma S et al (2004) Cyclooxygenase 2-dependent expression of survivin is critical for apoptosis resistance in non-small cell lung cancer. Cancer Res 64:6359–6362
76. Krysan K, Merchant FH, Zhu L et al (2004) COX-2-dependent stabilization of survivin in non-small cell lung cancer. FASEB J 18:206–208
77. Labrecque L, Nyalendo C, Langlois S et al (2004) Src-mediated tyrosine phosphorylation of caveolin-1 induces its association with membrane type 1 matrix metalloproteinase. J Biol Chem 279:52132–52140
78. Landesman-Bollag E, Romieu-Mourez R, Song DH et al (2001) Protein kinase CK2 in mammary gland tumorigenesis. Oncogene 20:3247–3257

79. Landesman-Bollag E, Song DH, Romieu-Mourez R et al (2001) Protein kinase CK2: signaling and tumorigenesis in the mammary gland. Mol Cell Biochem 227:153–165

80. Lavie Y, Fiucci G, Liscovitch M (1998) Up-regulation of caveolae and caveolar constituents in multidrug-resistant cancer cells. J Biol Chem 273:32380–32383

81. Lavie Y, Liscovitch M (2000) Changes in lipid and protein constituents of rafts and caveolae in multidrug resistant cancer cells and their functional consequences. Glycoconj J 17:253–259

82. Lee H, Volonte D, Galbiati F et al (2000) Constitutive and growth factor-regulated phosphorylation of caveolin-1 occurs at the same site (Tyr-14) in vivo: identification of a c-Src/Cav-1/Grb7 signaling cassette. Mol Endocrinol 14:1750–1775

83. Lee SW, Reimer CL, Oh P et al (1998) Tumor cell growth inhibition by caveolin re-expression in human breast cancer cells. Oncogene 16:1391–1397

84. Levina E, Oren M, Ben-Ze'ev A (2004) Downregulation of beta-catenin by p53 involves changes in the rate of beta-catenin phosphorylation and Axin dynamics. Oncogene 23:4444–4453

85. Li F, Ambrosini G, Chu EY et al (1998) Control of apoptosis and mitotic spindle checkpoint by survivin. Nature 396:580–584

86. Li J, Hassan GS, Williams TM et al (2005) Loss of caveolin-1 causes the hyper-proliferation of intestinal crypt stem cells, with increased sensitivity to whole body gamma-radiation. Cell Cycle 4:1817–1825

87. Li L, Ren C, Yang G et al (2009) Caveolin-1 promotes autoregulatory, Akt-mediated induction of cancer-promoting growth factors in prostate cancer cells. Mol Cancer Res 7:1781–1791

88. Li L, Yang G, Ebara S et al (2001) Caveolin-1 mediates testosterone-stimulated survival/clonal growth and promotes metastatic activities in prostate cancer cells. Cancer Res 61:4386–4392

89. Li S, Seitz R, Lisanti MP (1996) Phosphorylation of caveolin by src tyrosine kinases. The alpha-isoform of caveolin is selectively phosphorylated by v-Src in vivo. J Biol Chem 271:3863–3868

90. Li WP, Liu P, Pilcher BK et al (2001) Cell-specific targeting of caveolin-1 to caveolae, secretory vesicles, cytoplasm or mitochondria. J Cell Sci 114:1397–1408

91. Liou JY, Deng WG, Gilroy DW et al (2001) Colocalization and interaction of cyclooxygenase-2 with caveolin-1 in human fibroblasts. J Biol Chem 276:34975–34982

92. Liu C, Li Y, Semenov M et al (2002) Control of beta-catenin phosphorylation/degradation by a dual-kinase mechanism. Cell 108:837–847

93. Lu S, Gough AW, Bobrowski WF et al (1996) Transport properties are not altered across Caco-2 cells with heightened TEER despite underlying physiological and ultrastructural changes. J Pharm Sci 85:270–273

94. Ma DW, Seo J, Davidson LA et al (2004) n-3 PUFA alter caveolae lipid composition and resident protein localization in mouse colon. FASEB J 18:1040–1042

95. Maher MT, Flozak AS, Stocker AM et al (2009) Activity of the beta-catenin phosphodestruction complex at cell-cell contacts is enhanced by cadherin-based adhesion. J Cell Biol 186:219–228

96. Maier TJ, Janssen A, Schmidt R et al (2005) Targeting the beta-catenin/APC pathway: a novel mechanism to explain the cyclooxygenase-2-independent anticarcinogenic effects of celecoxib in human colon carcinoma cells. FASEB J 19:1353–1355

97. Mastick CC, Brady MJ, Saltiel AR (1995) Insulin stimulates the tyrosine phosphorylation of caveolin. J Cell Biol 129:1523–1531

98. Mastick CC, Saltiel AR (1997) Insulin-stimulated tyrosine phosphorylation of caveolin is specific for the differentiated adipocyte phenotype in 3T3-L1 cells. J Biol Chem 272:20706–20714

99. Mosimann C, Hausmann G, Basler K (2009) Beta-catenin hits chromatin: regulation of Wnt target gene activation. Nat Rev Mol Cell Biol 10:276–286

100. Nathke IS (2004) The adenomatous polyposis coli protein: the Achilles heel of the gut epithelium. Annu Rev Cell Dev Biol 20:337–366

101. Nusse R (2005) Wnt signaling in disease and in development. Cell Res 15:28–32
102. Okamoto T, Schlegel A, Scherer PE et al (1998) Caveolins, a family of scaffolding proteins for organizing "preassembled signaling complexes" at the plasma membrane. J Biol Chem 273:5419–5422
103. Orlichenko L, Huang B, Krueger E et al (2006) Epithelial growth factor-induced phosphorylation of caveolin 1 at tyrosine 14 stimulates caveolae formation in epithelial cells. J Biol Chem 281:4570–4579
104. Parat MO, Anand-Apte B, Fox PL (2003) Differential caveolin-1 polarization in endothelial cells during migration in two and three dimensions. Mol Biol Cell 14:3156–3168
105. Park DS, Cohen AW, Frank PG et al (2003) Caveolin-1 null (−/−) mice show dramatic reductions in life span. Biochemistry 42:15124–15131
106. Park JY, Pillinger MH, Abramson SB (2006) Prostaglandin E2 synthesis and secretion: the role of PGE2 synthases. Clin Immunol 119:229–240
107. Patlolla JM, Swamy MV, Raju J et al (2004) Overexpression of caveolin-1 in experimental colon adenocarcinomas and human colon cancer cell lines. Oncol Rep 11:957–963
108. Perrone G, Zagami M, Altomare V et al (2007) COX-2 localization within plasma membrane caveolae-like structures in human lobular intraepithelial neoplasia of the breast. Virchows Arch 451:1039–1045
109. Polakis P (2000) Wnt signaling and cancer. Genes Dev 14:1837–1851
110. Prescott SM, Fitzpatrick FA (2000) Cyclooxygenase-2 and carcinogenesis. Biochim Biophys Acta 1470:M69–M78
111. Quest AF, Gutierrez-Pajares JL, Torres VA (2008) Caveolin-1: an ambiguous partner in cell signalling and cancer. J Cell Mol Med 12:1130–1150
112. Quest AF, Leyton L, Parraga M (2004) Caveolins, caveolae, and lipid rafts in cellular transport, signaling, and disease. Biochem Cell Biol 82:129–144
113. Racine C, Belanger M, Hirabayashi H et al (1999) Reduction of caveolin 1 gene expression in lung carcinoma cell lines. Biochem Biophys Res Commun 255:580–586
114. Radtke F, Clevers H (2005) Self-renewal and cancer of the gut: two sides of a coin. Science 307:1904–1909
115. Razani B, Engelman JA, Wang XB et al (2001) Caveolin-1 null mice are viable but show evidence of hyperproliferative and vascular abnormalities. J Biol Chem 276:38121–38138
116. Razani B, Schlegel A, Lisanti MP (2000) Caveolin proteins in signaling, oncogenic transformation and muscular dystrophy. J Cell Sci 113(pt 12):2103–2109
117. Razani B, Woodman SE, Lisanti MP (2002) Caveolae: from cell biology to animal physiology. Pharmacol Rev 54:431–467
118. Reed JC (2001) The Survivin saga goes in vivo. J Clin Invest 108:965–969
119. Rodriguez DA, Tapia JC, Fernandez JG et al (2009) Caveolin-1-mediated suppression of cyclooxygenase-2 via a beta-catenin-Tcf/Lef-dependent transcriptional mechanism reduced prostaglandin E2 production and survivin expression. Mol Biol Cell 20:2297–2310
120. Sadot E, Conacci-Sorrell M, Zhurinsky J et al (2002) Regulation of S33/S37 phosphorylated beta-catenin in normal and transformed cells. J Cell Sci 115:2771–2780
121. Sanguinetti AR, Mastick CC (2003) c-Abl is required for oxidative stress-induced phosphorylation of caveolin-1 on tyrosine 14. Cell Signal 15:289–298
122. Santilman V, Baran J, Anand-Apte B et al (2007) Caveolin-1 polarization in transmigrating endothelial cells requires binding to intermediate filaments. Angiogenesis 10:297–305
123. Savage K, Lambros MB, Robertson D et al (2007) Caveolin 1 is overexpressed and amplified in a subset of basal-like and metaplastic breast carcinomas: a morphologic, ultrastructural, immunohistochemical, and in situ hybridization analysis. Clin Cancer Res 13:90–101
124. Scherer PE, Tang Z, Chun M et al (1995) Caveolin isoforms differ in their N-terminal protein sequence and subcellular distribution. Identification and epitope mapping of an isoform-specific monoclonal antibody probe. J Biol Chem 270:16395–16401
125. Seldin DC, Landesman-Bollag E, Farago M et al (2005) CK2 as a positive regulator of Wnt signalling and tumourigenesis. Mol Cell Biochem 274:63–67

126. Selga E, Morales C, Noe V et al (2008) Role of caveolin 1, E-cadherin, Enolase 2 and PKCalpha on resistance to methotrexate in human HT29 colon cancer cells. BMC Med Genomics 1:35

127. Shao J, Jung C, Liu C et al (2005) Prostaglandin E2 stimulates the beta-catenin/T cell factor-dependent transcription in colon cancer. J Biol Chem 280:26565–26572

128. Shao J, Lee SB, Guo H et al (2003) Prostaglandin E2 stimulates the growth of colon cancer cells via induction of amphiregulin. Cancer Res 63:5218–5223

129. Sloan EK, Ciocca DR, Pouliot N et al (2009) Stromal cell expression of caveolin-1 predicts outcome in breast cancer. Am J Pathol 174:2035–2043

130. Song DH, Dominguez I, Mizuno J et al (2003) CK2 phosphorylation of the armadillo repeat region of beta-catenin potentiates Wnt signaling. J Biol Chem 278:24018–24025

131. Song DH, Sussman DJ, Seldin DC (2000) Endogenous protein kinase CK2 participates in Wnt signaling in mammary epithelial cells. J Biol Chem 275:23790–23797

132. Sun XH, Flynn DC, Castranova V et al (2007) Identification of a novel domain at the N terminus of caveolin-1 that controls rear polarization of the protein and caveolae formation. J Biol Chem 282:7232–7241

133. Sun XH, Liu ZY, Chen H et al (2009) A conserved sequence in caveolin-1 is both necessary and sufficient for caveolin polarity and cell directional migration. FEBS Lett 583:3681–3689

134. Sun Y, Tang XM, Half E et al (2002) Cyclooxygenase-2 overexpression reduces apoptotic susceptibility by inhibiting the cytochrome c-dependent apoptotic pathway in human colon cancer cells. Cancer Res 62:6323–6328

135. Tahir SA, Park S, Thompson TC (2009) Caveolin-1 regulates VEGF-stimulated angiogenic activities in prostate cancer and endothelial cells. Cancer Biol Ther 8(23):2286–2296

136. Tahir SA, Yang G, Ebara S et al (2001) Secreted caveolin-1 stimulates cell survival/clonal growth and contributes to metastasis in androgen-insensitive prostate cancer. Cancer Res 61:3882–3885

137. Tapia JC, Torres VA, Rodriguez DA et al (2006) Casein kinase 2 (CK2) increases survivin expression via enhanced beta-catenin-T cell factor/lymphoid enhancer binding factor-dependent transcription. Proc Natl Acad Sci USA 103:15079–15084

138. Torres VA, Tapia JC, Rodriguez DA et al (2006) Caveolin-1 controls cell proliferation and cell death by suppressing expression of the inhibitor of apoptosis protein survivin. J Cell Sci 119:1812–1823

139. Torres VA, Tapia JC, Rodriguez DA et al (2007) E-cadherin is required for caveolin-1-mediated down-regulation of the inhibitor of apoptosis protein survivin via reduced beta-catenin-Tcf/Lef-dependent transcription. Mol Cell Biol 27:7703–7717

140. van Deurs B, Roepstorff K, Hommelgaard AM et al (2003) Caveolae: anchored, multifunctional platforms in the lipid ocean. Trends Cell Biol 13:92–100

141. Volonte D, Galbiati F, Pestell RG et al (2001) Cellular stress induces the tyrosine phosphory-lation of caveolin-1 (Tyr(14)) via activation of p38 mitogen-activated protein kinase and c-Src kinase. Evidence for caveolae, the actin cytoskeleton, and focal adhesions as mechanical sensors of osmotic stress. J Biol Chem 276:8094–8103

142. Wang S, Jones KA (2006) CK2 controls the recruitment of Wnt regulators to target genes in vivo. Curr Biol 16:2239–2244

143. Watabe M, Nagafuchi A, Tsukita S et al (1994) Induction of polarized cell-cell association and retardation of growth by activation of the E-cadherin-catenin adhesion system in a dispersed carcinoma line. J Cell Biol 127:247–256

144. Widelitz R (2005) Wnt signaling through canonical and non-canonical pathways: recent progress. Growth Factors 23:111–116

145. Wiechen K, Diatchenko L, Agoulnik A et al (2001) Caveolin-1 is down-regulated in human ovarian carcinoma and acts as a candidate tumor suppressor gene. Am J Pathol 159:1635–1643

146. Wiechen K, Sers C, Agoulnik A et al (2001) Down-regulation of caveolin-1, a candidate tumor suppressor gene, in sarcomas. Am J Pathol 158:833–839

147. Williams TM, Cheung MW, Park DS et al (2003) Loss of caveolin-1 gene expression accelerates the development of dysplastic mammary lesions in tumor-prone transgenic mice. Mol Biol Cell 14:1027–1042

148. Williams TM, Lisanti MP (2004) The caveolin proteins. Genome Biol 5:214
149. Williams TM, Lisanti MP (2005) Caveolin-1 in oncogenic transformation, cancer, and metastasis. Am J Physiol Cell Physiol 288:C494–C506
150. Witkiewicz AK, Dasgupta A, Sotgia F et al (2009) An absence of stromal caveolin-1 expression predicts early tumor recurrence and poor clinical outcome in human breast cancers. Am J Pathol 174:2023–2034
151. Xing Y, Clements WK, Le Trong I et al (2004) Crystal structure of a beta-catenin/APC complex reveals a critical role for APC phosphorylation in APC function. Mol Cell 15:523–533
152. Yamaguchi H, Takeo Y, Yoshida S et al (2009) Lipid rafts and caveolin-1 are required for invadopodia formation and extracellular matrix degradation by human breast cancer cells. Cancer Res 69:8594–8602
153. Yang G, Addai J, Wheeler TM et al (2007) Correlative evidence that prostate cancer cell-derived caveolin-1 mediates angiogenesis. Hum Pathol 38:1688–1695
154. Yang G, Truong LD, Timme TL et al (1998) Elevated expression of caveolin is associated with prostate and breast cancer. Clin Cancer Res 4:1873–1880
155. Zeng X, Tamai K, Doble B et al (2005) A dual-kinase mechanism for Wnt co-receptor phosphorylation and activation. Nature 438:873–877
156. Zhang H, Su L, Muller S et al (2008) Restoration of caveolin-1 expression suppresses growth and metastasis of head and neck squamous cell carcinoma. Br J Cancer 99:1684–1694
157. Zhang T, Otevrel T, Gao Z et al (2001) Evidence that APC regulates survivin expression: a possible mechanism contributing to the stem cell origin of colon cancer. Cancer Res 61:8664–8667

Chapter 3
Caveolin-1 and Pancreatic Ductal Adenocarcinoma

David W. Rittenhouse, Oeendree Mukherjee, Nathan G. Richards, Charles J. Yeo, Agnieszka K. Witkiewicz, and Jonathan R. Brody

Introduction: Pancreatic Ductal Adenocarcinoma

Even though tremendous resources have been poured into genome wide analyses of pancreatic cancer genomes, pancreatic ductal adenocarcinoma (PDA) still remains a devastating disease [1]. While being the eleventh most common malignancy in the western world, PDA ranks as the fourth leading cause of cancer-related deaths, with a dismal 5-year survival of less than 6% [2]. To underscore this point, the incidence of the disease nearly matches the mortality every year. In fact, it is estimated that in 2010, nearly 43,000 Americans were diagnosed with PDA with almost 37,000 people dying from disease-related complications [3]. At present, the only potential cure for PDA is surgical resection; however, only less than 20% of patients are resectable at the time of diagnosis [2].

The reason for this low percentage of patients meeting the operability criteria for resection is due, in part, to the indolent nature of PDA (i.e., the majority of patients present with locally advanced or metastatic disease). Based on these grim statistics, there is a dire need for a better molecular understanding of the etiology of this disease. Past work has proven that a series of genetic mutations such as *k-ras*, *SMAD4*, and *p53* are critical for pancreatic tumorigenesis [4–6]. Jones et al. further demonstrated that only a small fraction of overexpressed genes, via serial analysis of gene expression

D.W. Rittenhouse • O. Mukherjee • N.G. Richards • C.J. Yeo
Department of Surgery, Jefferson Pancreas, Biliary and Related Cancer Center,
and Kimmel Cancer Center, Thomas Jefferson University, Philadelphia, PA, USA

A.K. Witkiewicz • J.R. Brody (✉)
Department of Surgery, Jefferson Pancreas, Biliary and Related Cancer Center,
and Kimmel Cancer Center, Thomas Jefferson University, Philadelphia, PA, USA

Department of Pathology, Thomas Jefferson University, Philadelphia, PA, USA
e-mail: jonathan.brody@jefferson.edu

I. Mercier et al. (eds.), *Caveolins in Cancer Pathogenesis, Prevention and Therapy*,
Current Cancer Research, DOI 10.1007/978-1-4614-1001-0_3,
© Springer Science+Business Media, LLC 2012

(SAGE) in PDA, could be explained by mutations alone [1]. This finding suggests that exploring other molecular events that disrupt the 12 identified core signaling pathways in PDA may be critical for our further molecular understanding and ultimately for future targeted treatment of this disease [1].

Caveolin-1

Caveolae are flask-shaped invaginations of the cellular plasma membrane that were first observed by electron microscopy in the 1950s [7]. Caveolin-1 (Cav-1) is the most prominent protein component of caveolar membranes; however, many important signaling molecules are localized in caveolae including the Src family of kinases, H-ras, protein kinase C, the epidermal growth factor receptor (EGFR), the platelet-derived growth factor receptor (PDGFR), and endothelial nitric oxide synthase (eNOS). Structurally, Caveolins are integral membrane proteins consisting of three isoforms of which Cav-1 (22-kDa) and -2 (20-kDa) are ubiquitously expressed [8]. Functionally, Cav-1 is essential for caveolae-related endo- and exocytosis transport processes and intracellular signal transduction. In caveolae, caveolins oligomerize and associate with cholesterol and sphingolipids in distinct areas of the cell membrane. Commonly, signaling proteins are activated by conformational changes upon release from caveolins. For instance, caveolins contain a specific inhibitory binding domain called caveolin scaffolding domain (CSD), which allows the interaction with different signaling proteins. Functionally, Cav-1 plays an important role in signal transduction, membrane trafficking, and cholesterol transport [9].

Caveolin-1 and the Proliferation of Cancer

Although Cav-1 has been shown in multiple settings to be critical for pancreatic tumorigenesis, the exact role of Cav-1 in pancreatic tumor cell promotion and survival is unclear. Recent data show its importance in a newly described tumorigenic mechanism involving the tumor microenvironment called the "reverse Warburg effect" [10]. Many previous studies suggest that Cav-1 is a tumor suppressor gene. For example, down-regulation of Cav-1 expression was observed in breast, lung, colon, and ovarian cancers [11–13]. Ectopic expression of Cav-1 in transformed normal cells and tumor cell lines inhibited cell growth in vitro and tumorigenesis in vivo. Further, Sunaga et al. reported that Cav-1 acted like a tumor suppressor gene in small cell lung cancer, whereas in nonsmall cell lung cancer it is required for cell survival and growth [14, 15]. In contrast, other studies have reported that Cav-1 expression was up-regulated in human cancers, including prostate cancer and esophageal squamous cell carcinoma [16, 17]. These results suggest that the roles of Cav-1 may vary depending upon the type of tumor or the experimental setting.

Duxbury et al. shed some light on the mechanism through which Cav-1 influences cancer cell properties (i.e., extracellular signaling events and malignant cellular behavior) [18]. Cross-linking of carcinoembryonic antigen-related cell adhesion molecule 6 (CEACAM6), a prominent glycosylphosphatidylinositol (GPI) anchored cell surface protein that is expressed in a variety of human malignancies, activates c-Src tyrosine kinase in a Cav-1-dependent manner [18]. CEACAM6 crosslinking decreases Cav-1-induced dissociation of the c-Src tyrosine kinase from the CEAC-AM6-Cav1 membrane complex and activation of focal adhesion kinase (FAK) by phosphorylation. As a result, anchorage-independent cell survival is achieved, resulting in cellular resistance to anoikis (a form of apoptosis).

In addition to Src-dependent pathways, Cav-1 activation also controls intracellular signaling via Akt, a serine/threonine kinase. Li et al. showed that the mechanical force from increased glomerular hydrostatic pressure leads to Cav-1 phosphorylation, which activates EGFR [19]. EGFR activation of Akt leads to activation and increased collagen-1 production [19]. Additionally, Li et al. showed that Cav-1 inhibits protein phosphatases 1 and 2A and activates phosphatidylinositol-3-OH kinase (PI3-K), which leads to increased Akt expression and increased survival of prostate cancer cells [20]. These studies may help to explain how increased Cav-1 expression is associated with aggressive stages in malignancies such as colon, bladder, ovarian, and pancreatic.

Caveolin-1 in the Pathogenesis of Pancreatic Ductal Adenocarcinoma

It is still unclear whether Cav-1 overexpression plays a role in pancreatic cancer cell growth as a tumor promoter or suppressor. Further, ongoing studies will reveal the role of Cav-1 in the pancreatic tumor microenvironment and accordingly, its role in the recent proposal of the "reverse Warburg effect" in PDA development and survival mechanisms [10]. Yang et al. generated a transgenic mouse model that constitutively overexpressed Cav-1 under the regulation of mouse mammary tumor virus (MMTV) promoter, i.e., MMTV-Cav-1 transgenic mice [21]. The transgenic mice displayed defective morphologic features, mainly in epithelial cells of multiple exocrine organs. These results indicate that Cav-1 overexpression may cause organ-specific, age-related epithelial disorders, and suggest the potential for increased susceptibility to carcinogenesis [21]. As an important glandular organ exhibiting both endocrine and exocrine functionalities, the pancreas could be highly susceptible to the carcinogenetic effects of Cav-1. In this mouse model, the investigators demonstrated that overexpresion of Cav-1 led to pancreatic acinar cells with decreased eosinophilic zygogen granules when compared with their control littermates without Cav-1 overexpression [21].

Additionally, Cav-1 has also been shown to regulate PDA tumorigenesis through the regulation of matrix metalloproteinases (MMPs). MMPs are a family of proteolytic enzymes with different substrate specificities responsible for the breakdown of extracellular matrix [22]. As a gelatinase subgroup of MMPs, both MMP2 and MMP9 degrade type IV collagen and are believed to play an important role in pancreatic tumor cell invasion [22]. Several experimental models have suggested that expression of MMP2 and MMP9 were both positively correlated with aggressiveness of some pancreatic carcinoma cells in vitro, and in preclinical in vivo mice models [23–25]. Complementary to these studies, Bramhall et al. reported that MMP2 was up-regulated in pancreatitis and PDA, whereas it was absent in normal pancreas cells [26]. In addition, Kuniyasu et al. reported MMP2 expression was more abundant at the invasive front of the tumor, rather than in the tumor center in PDA [22]. Koshiba et al. supported this work by showing that overexpression of MMP2 was positively correlated with lymph node metastases and distant metastases in PDA [27]. Combining this work, Williams et al. reported that overexpression of Cav-1 in metastatic breast cancer cells reduced cell invasion capacity, which might be mediated partly through inhibition of MMP2 and MMP9 activities [28]. Although these studies support the notion that Cav-1 directly regulates the activity of MMP2, it remains unknown whether other signaling molecules participate in this process.

As an example, Han et al. recently reported on the regulatory role of Cav-1 on MMPs in pancreatic cancer cells [29]. In their study, it was found that Cav-1 expression inversely correlated with the invasion of PDA cell lines BxPc3 and SW1990 using a cell invasion assay [29]. The number of SW1990 invasive cells was decreased by 3.8-fold when comparing Cav-1 overexpressing cells with controls. Inversely, knockdown of Cav-1 with siRNA oligonucleotides in BxPc3 cells led to a 2.7-fold increase in the number of invasive cells, while the inhibition of the extracellular signal-regulated kinase (Erk) signal molecule reduced EGF-induced MMP2 and MMP9 activity. These data suggest that there are most likely many factors affecting the regulatory role of Cav-1 on MMP's ability to enhance PDA tumorigenesis.

Cav-1 also has a defined inhibitory role on pancreatic cancer cell growth. One of the pathways in which Cav-1 inhibits PDA tumorigenesis is the EGFR-mitogen-activated protein kinase (MAPK) signaling pathway. Han et al. explored the mechanism of Cav-1 regulation of the EGFR-MAPK pathway in regards to pancreatic cancer growth [30]. Results of their study suggested that overexpression of Cav-1 inhibited the proliferation of pancreatic carcinoma cells both in vitro and in vivo (i.e., Panc 1 cell growth in nude mice).

Cav-1 has also been shown to play an inhibitory role in PDA growth through the interaction with Rho GTPases. Rho GTPases are small monomeric molecules that are typically involved in actin cytoskeleton re-arrangement during cellular migration [31]. RhoC GTPase is a member of the GTPase subfamily that is associated with highly aggressive and metastatic tumors including PDA [31]. Cav-1 expression inhibits RhoC GTPase activation and subsequent activation of the p38 MAPK pathway in primary PDA cells, thus restricting the migratory and invasive potential of these cells. Lin et al. studied the effect of Cav-1 on PDA cellular migration and invasion. This study analyzed ten PDA cell lines and compared Cav-1 expression with PDA cell lines derived from metastatic cells. Elevated Cav-1 expression was found in BxPc3 and MiaPaca2 cell lines (derived from primary PDA tumors) and low Cav-1 expression was found in HPAF1, Capan1, Capan2, and ASPC1 (derived from meta-static PDA cells or cells in malignant ascitic fluid). Mechanistically, the study found that Cav-1 expression suppresses Rhoc GTPase activation and RhoC-mediated cellular migration and invasion [32]. The investigators demonstrated that loss of Cav-1 expression leads to increased RhoC activation by favoring the p38 MAPK pathway, which results in cellular migration and invasion. In contrast, loss of Cav-1 expression leads to RhoC-mediated migration and invasion in metastatic PDA cell lines [32]. Also, expression of Cav-1 was noted to favor activation of the p42/p44 Erk pathway, perhaps promoting growth and survival of the primary PDA cell lines. This might underscore the presence of a differential expression of Cav-1 during the complex tumorigenesis process, where the overexpression of Cav-1 may lead to increased tumor growth, and conversely a switch to decreased Cav-1 expression may make a cell more likely to metastasize [32].

Caveolin-1 as a Biomarker in Pancreatic Ductal Adenocarcinoma

Suzuoki and et al. studied the role of epithelial Cav-1 expression as a prognostic marker for PDA in 79 patients undergoing surgery [33]. The 3-year survival rate following surgical resection in the Cav-1 negative group was 33.8%, while the 3-year survival rate in the Cav-1 positive group was only 4.8%. Positive Cav-1 expression was correlated with larger tumor diameter ($p=0.0079$), histopathologic grade ($p=0.0272$), and poor prognosis ($p=0.0008$). Upon multivariate analysis with a Cox proportional hazards model, positive Cav-1 expression was shown to be an independent negative predictor for survival ($p=0.0358$) [33]. These results imply a role for Cav-1 expression in determining the prognosis of patients with resected pancreatic cancer and also support the role of Cav-1 as a biomarker.

Tanase et al. reported that Cav-1 expression was positively correlated with tumor diameter, histopathologic grade, and other tumor biomarkers [34]. Western blot analysis confirmed the overexpression of Cav-1 in PDA tumors when compared with peritumoral tissue. Cav-1 expression in tumor tissues was correlated with both Ki-67 and p53 expressions. Overexpression of Cav-1 was associated with tumor size, grade, stage, and increased serum level of CA 19-9 (CA 19-9 is a nonspecific biomarker for PDA) in PDA patients [34].

We have demonstrated that Cav-1 expression correlated with poor differentiation status of PDA tumor and also correlated with fatty acid synthase (FASN) expression (Fig. 3.1) [35]. FASN is a lipogenic enzyme, which catalyzes the terminal steps of fatty acid biosynthesis [36]. Like Cav-1, FASN has been shown to be dysregulated in a number of cancers such as breast and prostate, where higher expression levels of FASN have been correlated with advanced tumor stage and poor prognosis [35, 37]. Expression of both Cav-1 and FASN has a positive correlation with malignant disease in PDA (Fig. 3.1). Conversely, a significant survival advantage was found in patients with low expression of Cav-1 [37]. Specifically, Cav-1 and FASN expression are absent in precursor lesions of PDA, pancreatic intraepithelial neoplasia (PanINs), and normal pancreatic ducts, but both may be elevated in PDA. The fact that Cav-1

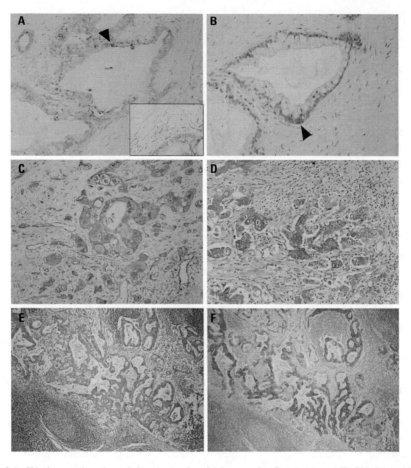

Fig. 3.1 Weak cytoplasmic staining (*arrowheads*) is seen for Cav-1 (**a**) and FASN (**b**) in histologic slides of a well-differentiated PDA. Strong cytoplasmic staining is seen for Cav-1 (**c**, **e**) and FASN (**d**, **f**) in histologic slides of a poorly-differentiated PDA and lymph node metastases (**e**, **f**), respectively [35]

and FASN are lost in PanINs, but elevated in PDA, suggest that Cav-1 overexpression is a late event in the progression of PDA tumorigenesis (Figs. 3.1 and 3.2). There is a strong positive correlation between expression of both Cav-1 and FASN with histologic grade and tumor stage in PDA [35]. Moreover, Cav-1 has been shown to be required for upregulation of FASN [38]. Further studies are necessary to determine the molecular mechanisms by which Cav-1 acts in promoting a metastatic phenotype, but upregulation of FASN could represent one possible mechanism. Further evaluation may validate FASN as a target for pancreatic cancer treatment, as a number of studies have shown successful pharmacologic blockade through various inhibitors of FASN is cytostatic and cytotoxic to tumor cells [37].

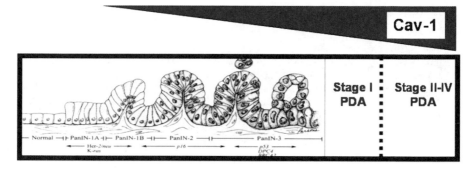

Fig. 3.2 Progression model of tumorigenesis in PDA displaying low Cav-1 expression in precursor lesions and high Cav-1 expression in PDA (primary tumors)

Caveolin-1 as a Targeted Therapy in Pancreatic Ductal Adenocarcinoma

Targeting strategies against central regulatory molecules involved in PDA tumorigenesis have the potential to improve cancer therapy and patient survival. Here are a few examples of pre-clinical experiments that underscore this point. Cordes et al. have demonstrated that human pancreatic cancer cells can be rendered sensitive to ionizing radiation therapy by means of Cav-1 knockdown in two-dimensional (2D) grown cell culture [39]. Hehlgans et al. recently showed that Cav-1 could be used as a potential target molecule in human PDA cells in a 3D cell culture model. In these studies, Cav-1 was overexpressed into MiaPaca2 and Panc1 PDA cell lines, which increased cell survival after treatment with radiation. In contrast, silencing of Cav-1 expression via siRNA oligonucleotides made cells more radiosensitive [40]. Based on this body of work, knowledge of the Cav-1 expression in a patient's resected tumor sample may prove useful as a predictive biomarker for their response to radiation therapy. Furthermore, for patients with elevated Cav-1 expression, Cav-1 siRNA could someday be targeted to the tumor bed via nanoparticle therapy or small compounds to silence Cav-1 function, thereby making the tumor more susceptible to radiation therapy [41].

In conclusion, knowledge of Cav-1 expression in resected or biopsied specimens may also prove to be a useful index of predictor of response to adjuvant therapy for patients with an already high risk of poor prognosis [35]. Yet, the most exciting therapeutic intervention of Cav-1 biology in pancreatic cancer cells may lie with targeting the direct relationship of Cav-1 with an important tumor promoting and survival mechanism involving the reverse Warburg effect (refer to Chapter 7 for more information) [10]. Further work in PDA preclinical models and patient samples will provide greater insight into the usefulness of Cav-1 as a target and tool for optimizing the treatment of pancreatic cancer.

References

1. Jones S, Zhang X, Parsons DW, Lin JC, Leary RJ, Angenendt P, Mankoo P, Carter H, Kamiyama H, Jimeno A, Hong SM, Fu B, Lin MT, Calhoun ES, Kamiyama M, Walter K, Nikolskaya T, Nikolsky Y, Hartigan J, Smith DR, Hidalgo M, Leach SD, Klein AP, Jaffee EM, Goggins M, Maitra A, Iacobuzio-Donahue C, Eshleman JR, Kern SE, Hruban RH, Karchin R, Papadopoulos N, Parmigiani G, Vogelstein B, Velculescu VE, Kinzler KW (2008) Core signaling pathways in human pancreatic cancers revealed by global genomic analyses. Science 321:1801–1806
2. Hidalgo M (2010) Pancreatic cancer. N Engl J Med 362:1605–1617
3. National Cancer Institute (2011) Pancreatic Cancer. http://www.cancer.gov/cancertopics/types/pancreatic
4. Smit VT, Boot AJ, Smits AM, Fleuren GJ, Cornelisse CJ, Bos JL (1988) KRAS codon 12 mutations occur very frequently in pancreatic adenocarcinomas. Nucleic Acids Res 16:7773–7782
5. Sohn TA, Su GH, Ryu B, Yeo CJ, Kern SE (2001) High-throughput drug screening of the DPC4 tumor-suppressor pathway in human pancreatic cancer cells. Ann Surg 233:696–703
6. Barton CM, Staddon SL, Hughes CM, Hall PA, O'Sullivan C, Kloppel G, Theis B, Russell RC, Neoptolemos J, Williamson RC et al (1991) Abnormalities of the p53 tumour suppressor gene in human pancreatic cancer. Br J Cancer 64:1076–1082
7. Liu J, Wang XB, Park DS, Lisanti MP (2002) Caveolin-1 expression enhances endothelial capillary tubule formation. J Biol Chem 277:10661–10668
8. Williams TM, Cheung MW, Park DS, Razani B, Cohen AW, Muller WJ, Di Vizio D, Chopra NG, Pestell RG, Lisanti MP (2003) Loss of caveolin-1 gene expression accelerates the development of dysplastic mammary lesions in tumor-prone transgenic mice. Mol Biol Cell 14:1027–1042
9. Couet J, Sargiacomo M, Lisanti MP (1997) Interaction of a receptor tyrosine kinase, EGF-R, with caveolins. Caveolin binding negatively regulates tyrosine and serine/threonine kinase activities. J Biol Chem 272:30429–30438
10. Bonuccelli G, Whitaker-Menezes D, Castello-Cros R, Pavlides S, Pestell RG, Fatatis A, Witkiewicz AK, Heiden MG, Migneco G, Chiavarina B, Frank PG, Capozza F, Flomenberg N, Martinez-Outschoorn UE, Sotgia F, Lisanti MP (2010) The reverse Warburg effect: glycolysis inhibitors prevent the tumor promoting effects of caveolin-1 deficient cancer associated fibroblasts. Cell Cycle 9:1960–1971
11. Sloan EK, Stanley KL, Anderson RL (2004) Caveolin-1 inhibits breast cancer growth and metastasis. Oncogene 23:7893–7897
12. Bender FC, Reymond MA, Bron C, Quest AF (2000) Caveolin-1 levels are down-regulated in human colon tumors, and ectopic expression of caveolin-1 in colon carcinoma cell lines reduces cell tumorigenicity. Cancer Res 60:5870–5878
13. Wiechen K, Diatchenko L, Agoulnik A, Scharff KM, Schober H, Arlt K, Zhumabayeva B, Siebert PD, Dietel M, Schafer R, Sers C (2001) Caveolin-1 is down-regulated in human ovarian carcinoma and acts as a candidate tumor suppressor gene. Am J Pathol 159:1635 1643
14. Sunaga N, Miyajima K, Suzuki M, Sato M, White MA, Ramirez RD, Shay JW, Gazdar AF, Minna JD (2004) Different roles for caveolin-1 in the development of non-small cell lung cancer versus small cell lung cancer. Cancer Res 64:4277–4285
15. Engelman JA, Zhang XL, Lisanti MP (1998) Genes encoding human caveolin-1 and -2 are co-localized to the D7S522 locus (7q31.1), a known fragile site (FRA7G) that is frequently deleted in human cancers. FEBS Lett 436:403–410
16. Yang G, Truong LD, Wheeler TM, Thompson TC (1999) Caveolin-1 expression in clinically confined human prostate cancer: a novel prognostic marker. Cancer Res 59:5719–5723
17. Han SE, Park KH, Lee G, Huh YJ, Min BM (2004) Mutation and aberrant expression of Caveolin-1 in human oral squamous cell carcinomas and oral cancer cell lines. Int J Oncol 24:435–440
18. Duxbury MS, Ito H, Ashley SW, Whang EE (2004) CEACAM6 cross-linking induces caveolin-1-dependent, Src-mediated focal adhesion kinase phosphorylation in BxPC3 pancreatic adenocarcinoma cells. J Biol Chem 279:23176–23182

19. Li L, Ren CH, Tahir SA, Ren C, Thompson TC (2003) Caveolin-1 maintains activated Akt in prostate cancer cells through scaffolding domain binding site interactions with and inhibition of serine/threonine protein phosphatases PP1 and PP2A. Mol Cell Biol 23:9389–9404
20. Li. L, Ren CH, Tahir SA, RenC, Thompson TC (2003) Caveolin-1 maintains activated Akt in prostate cancer cells through scaffolding domain binding site interactions with and inhibition of serine/threonine protein phosphatases PP1 and PP2A. Mol Cell Biol 23(24):9389–9404
21. Yang G, Park S, Cao G, Goltsov A, Ren C, Truong LD, Demavo F, Thompson TC (2010) MMTV promoter-regulated caveolin-1 overexpression yields defective parenchymal epithelia in multiple exocrine organs of transgenic mice. Exp Mol Pathol 89(1):9–19
22. Kuniyasu H, Ellis LM, Evans DB, Abbruzzese JL, Fenoglio CJ, Bucana CD, Cleary KR, Tahara E, Fidler IJ (1999) Relative expression of E-cadherin and type IV collagenase genes predicts disease outcome in patients with resectable pancreatic carcinoma. Clin Cancer Res 5:25–33
23. Haq M, Shafii A, Zervos EE, Rosemurgy AS (2000) Addition of matrix metalloproteinase inhibition to conventional cytotoxic therapy reduces tumor implantation and prolongs survival in a murine model of human pancreatic cancer. Cancer Res 60:3207–3211
24. Jimenez RE, Hartwig W, Antoniu BA, Compton CC, Warshaw AL (2000) Fernandez-Del Castillo C. Effect of matrix metalloproteinase inhibition on pancreatic cancer invasion and metastasis: an additive strategy for cancer control. Ann Surg 231:644–654
25. Zervos EE, Shafii AE, Rosemurgy AS (1999) Matrix metalloproteinase (MMP) inhibition selectively decreases type II MMP activity in a murine model of pancreatic cancer. J Surg Res 81:65–68
26. Bramhall SR (1997) The matrix metalloproteinases and their inhibitors in pancreatic cancer. From molecular science to a clinical application. Int J Pancreatol 21:1–12
27. Koshiba T, Hosotani R, Wada M, Miyamoto Y, Fujimoto K, Lee JU, Doi R, Arii S, Imamura M (1998) Involvement of matrix metalloproteinase-2 activity in invasion and metastasis of pancreatic carcinoma. Cancer 82:642–650
28. Williams TM, Medina F, Badano I, Hazan RB, Hutchinson J, Muller WJ, Chopra NG, Scherer PE, Pestell RG, Lisanti MP (2004) Caveolin-1 gene disruption promotes mammary tumorigenesis and dramatically enhances lung metastasis in vivo. Role of Cav-1 in cell invasiveness and matrix metalloproteinase (MMP-2/9) secretion. J Biol Chem 279:51630–51646
29. Han F, Zhu HG (2010) Caveolin-1 regulating the invasion and expression of matrix metalloproteinase (MMPs) in pancreatic carcinoma cells. J Surg Res 159:443–450
30. Han F, Gu D, Chen Q, Zhu H (2009) Caveolin-1 acts as a tumor suppressor by down-regulating epidermal growth factor receptor-mitogen-activated protein kinase signaling pathway in pancreatic carcinoma cell lines. Pancreas 38:766–774
31. Raftopoulou M, Hall A (2004) Cell migration:Rho GTPases lead the way. Dev Biol 265:23–32
32. Lin M, DiVito MM, Merajver SD, Boyanapalli M, van Golen KL (2005) Regulation of pancreatic cancer cell migration and invasion by RhoC GTPase and caveolin-1. Mol Cancer 4:21
33. Suzuoki M, Miyamoto M, Kato K, Hiraoka K, Oshikiri T, Nakakubo Y, Fukunaga A, Shichinohe T, Shinohara T, Itoh T, Kondo S, Katoh H (2002) Impact of caveolin-1 expression on prognosis of pancreatic ductal adenocarcinoma. Br J Cancer 87:1140–1144
34. Tanase CP, Dima S, Mihai M, Raducan E, Nicolescu MI, Albulescu L, Voiculescu B, Dumitrascu T, Cruceru LM, Leabu M, Popescu I, Hinescu ME (2009) Caveolin-1 overexpression correlates with tumour progression markers in pancreatic ductal adenocarcinoma. J Mol Histol 40:23–29
35. Witkiewicz AK, Nguyen KH, Dasgupta A, Kennedy EP, Yeo CJ, Lisanti MP, Brody JR (2008) Co-expression of fatty acid synthase and caveolin-1 in pancreatic ductal adenocarcinoma: implications for tumor progression and clinical outcome. Cell Cycle 7:3021–3025
36. Wakil SJ (1989) Fatty acid synthase, a proficient multifunctional enzyme. Biochemistry 28:4523–4530
37. Kuhajda FP (2006) Fatty acid synthase and cancer: new application of an old pathway. Cancer Res 66:5977–5980
38. Di Vizio D, Sotgia F, Williams TM, Hassan GS, Capozza F, Frank PG, Pestell RG, Loda M, Freeman MR, Lisanti MP (2007) Caveolin-1 is required for the upregulation of fatty acid synthase (FASN), a tumor promoter, during prostate cancer progression. Cancer Biol Ther 6:1263–1268

39. Cordes N, Frick S, Brunner TB, Pilarsky C, Grutzmann R, Sipos B, Kloppel G, McKenna WG, Bernhard EJ (2007) Human pancreatic tumor cells are sensitized to ionizing radiation by knockdown of caveolin-1. Oncogene 26:6851–6862
40. Hehlgans S, Eke I, Storch K, Haase M, Baretton GB, Cordes N (2009) Caveolin-1 mediated radioresistance of 3D grown pancreatic cancer cells. Radiother Oncol 92:362–370
41. Showalter SL, Huang YH, Witkiewicz A, Costantino CL, Yeo CJ, Green JJ, Langer R, Anderson DG, Sawicki JA, Brody JR (2008) Nanoparticulate delivery of diphtheria toxin DNA effectively kills Mesothelin expressing pancreatic cancer cells. Cancer Biol Ther 7:1584–1590

Chapter 4
Caveolin-1 in Brain Tumors

Rebecca Senetta and Paola Cassoni

Rapid Focus on Caveolin-1

Caveolin-1 (cav-1) is a multifunctional membrane protein localized in invaginations of the plasma membrane, called *caveolae*. Cav-1 participates in numerous cell functions such as cell signaling, trafficking, transport, compartmentalization, and motility, interferes with cell cycle regulation, and may contribute to multidrug resistance [1, 2]. In addition, cav-1 can positively and negatively affect tumor progression. In fact, contradictory evidences highlighted a role for cav-1 as either a tumor suppressor or promoter [3, 4]. Based on molecular and genetic evidences, the "*caveolae signaling hypothesis*" suggested *caveolae* as sites of complex regulation of signal modulation transduction involved in different disease processes [5]. Several authors [6–15] determined the expression of cav-1 in various solid tumors alternatively supporting its role in tumor progression or suppression. However, the role of cav-1 in brain tumor onset and progression still remains elusive.

Caveolin-1 in the Normal Brain

In normal brain tissue, cav-1 was first identified in glial cells [16–18] as well as in brain vessels [19]. In fact, Cameron et al. [16] identified *caveolae* and cav-1 immunoreactivity at the cell surface of cultured type 1 rat astrocytes and assumed the possibility of a cav-1 regulation during brain development. Ikezu et al. [17] later demonstrated the presence of at least two isoforms of caveolins in primary cultures of rat astrocytes. Moreover, Virgintino et al. [19] showed a rich caveolar compartment in brain endothelial cells, pericytes, and astrocytes *in vivo*.

R. Senetta • P. Cassoni (✉)
Department of Biomedical Sciences and Human Oncology, University of Turin, Turin, Italy
e-mail: paola.cassoni@unito.it

I. Mercier et al. (eds.), *Caveolins in Cancer Pathogenesis, Prevention and Therapy*,
Current Cancer Research, DOI 10.1007/978-1-4614-1001-0_4,
© Springer Science+Business Media, LLC 2012

Caveolin-1 in the Neoplastic Brain: Inputs from Cell Lines and Primary Tumors of Astrocytic Origin

The hypothesis that cav-1 acts as a tumor suppressor [7, 10, 20–23] is consistent with data showing that the cav-1 gene mapped to a fragile region (7q31.1), frequently deleted in tumors [24–27]. According to this evidence and to previous results in solid tumors, cav-1 expression was expected to be reduced in glioma cells. However, the first published data investigating the expression of cav-1 in neoplastic glial cells, conducted on the rat C6 astrocytoma cell line [28], demonstrated the maintenance of cav-1 expression. Furthermore, a differential temporal pattern of caveolin gene expression during phenotypic differentiation of C6 cells was later reported [29]. The results obtained in rat glioma cells were confirmed and expanded to human astroglioma cell lines a few years later. In fact, two rat astrocytoma-derived cell lines as well as five human glioblastoma cell lines showed cav-1 positivity, with localization pattern, density-insolubility properties, and buoyant density equivalent to that detected in non-transformed cultured astrocytes [30]. Moreover, immuno-fluorescence analyses demonstrated that the pattern of cav-1 expression was similar in all human glioblastoma cell lines, consisting in a punctuate membrane positivity associated with a diffuse cellular positivity with a reinforced localization in peri-nuclear and golgian regions. Despite what was reported in a previous study on breast carcinoma [31] and recently confirmed with additional functional data [32–34], no mutations of the cav-1 sequence were observed in human glioma cells. In fact, the nucleotide sequence from the cav-1 cDNA obtained from each human glioma cell line revealed a 100% identity to the human cav-1 genomic sequence [30]. Similarly, no post-translational modifications were observed. The study by Cameron et al. [30] thus provided a convincing demonstration that cav-1 expression was not sufficient to prevent the acquisition of a transformed phenotype in glial-derived tumors. Other authors reported that cav-1 immunodetection in human astrocytic brain tumors did not differ from normal brain [35]. In addition, a similar cav-1 expression was observed in tissue homogenates obtained from human astroglial tumors of different grades (I to IV), despite a grade-variable expression of caveolae-associated Rho GTPases [35]. However, the above quoted studies [35, 36] evaluated the presence of cav-1 through in vitro systems or in tissue homogenates. Therefore, no data were available on the effective distribution of cav-1 within the specific cell types present in primary brain tumors of different glial origin and grade.

Clarification of the effective distribution of cav-1 in glial-derived tumors came from one of our recent study, which first showed, in a series of 64 glial tumors, that cav-1 expression in human brain tumors varied depending on their origin (astrocytic vs oligodendroglial cells) and grade [37] (Figs. 4.1 and 4.2). Such evidence was confirmed in vitro by immunofluorescence analyses of established glioblastoma cell lines and primary cultures derived from glial tumors [37].

In astrocytic-derived gliomas, an intense cav-1 immunoreactivity is present at the membrane in high grade tumors with variable percentages of positive cells from a case to another. In contrast to this membranous pattern of staining, low grade

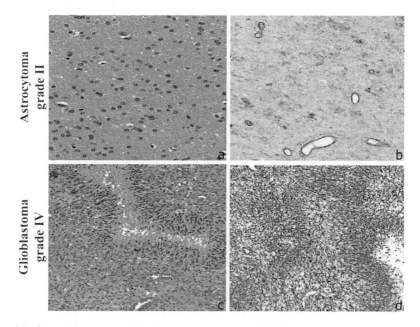

Fig. 4.1 Cav-1 immunoreactivity in astrocytic tumors of different grades. (**a**) Representative histological section of a grade II diffuse astrocytoma (H&E, original magnification: 20×) which shows (**b**) a specific cytoplasmic/dot-like perinuclear cav-1 staining pattern (original magnification: 20×). (**c**) Representative histological section of a glioblastoma (grade IV) showing an area of typical peri-necrotic palisade (H&E, original magnification: 20×). (**d**) Both the palisade and non-palisade neoplastic cells display strong and diffuse cav-1 staining with a predominant membrane pattern (original magnification: 20×)

gliomas display a finely granular matrix and/or cytoplasmic dot-like cav-1 immuno-reactivity (Fig. 4.1). Although being considered as low-grade gliomas, grade II gemistocytic gliomas are an exception to this rule, showing an intense membrane and cytoplasmic cav-1 staining throughout almost the totality of neoplastic cells. As a general consideration, the prevalent membrane cav-1 immunoreactivity observed in high grade gliomas compared with low grade tumors suggests that a more "struc-tured" cav-1 expression correlates with increased aggressiveness. In glioblastoma cells, cav-1 has been reported to colocalize with EGFR, and EGFR sequestration within *caveolae* seems to modulate EGFR-signaling and its role in glial cell transformation [36]. Therefore, the membrane cav-1 pattern observed in high grade gliomas but not in diffuse grade II astrocytomas seems more "functional" in hosting EGFR than the dot-like positivity. However, Barresi et al. [38] did not observe any correlation between EGFR overexpression and cav-1 positivity in a series of glio-blastomas but instead reported that high cav-1 expression was significantly associated with p53 overexpression. The EGFR and cav-1 relationship in brain tumors, which is extremely challenging under multiple points of view, needs further clarification and will be discussed later.

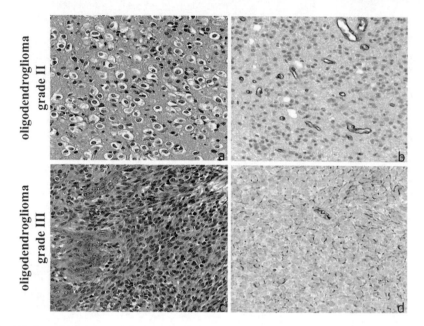

Fig. 4.2 Cav-1 immunoreactivity in grade II oligodendrogliomas and grade III anaplastic oligoden-drogliomas. (**a**) Representative histological section of a grade II oligodendroglioma (H&E, original magnification: 20×) and (**b**) its correspondent cav-1 immunostaining show a lack of cav-1 expression in neoplastic cells; cav-1 positivity is limited to the vessel wall which represents an internal positive control (original magnification: 20×). (**c**) Representative histological section of a grade III anaplastic oligodendroglioma (H&E, original magnification: 20×) in which (**d**) a fragmented cav-1 membrane positivity is evident (original magnification: 20×)

As mentioned above, the "alternate" dot-like cav-1 staining typical of grade II astrocytomas appears inadequate for its association with EGFR. Interestingly, in a recent study by Mercier et al. [34], two distinct patterns of cav-1 immunostaining were described in breast carcinomas, and proved to be associated with either the most common cav-1 mutation (P132L) (punctuate pattern) or the wild type protein (diffuse pattern of staining). Perinuclear accumulation of cav-1 was observed in well differentiated and ER-positive breast carcinomas. Such observations suggest that, similarly to what reported in breast cancer, the dot-like cav-1 staining detected in low grade astrocytomas could represent a mutated cav-1 isoform. The dot-like cav-1 staining observed in low grade astrocytomas could therefore result from a compensatory up-regulation, due to a loss-of-function or a dominant-negative mutation, and correspond to the accumulation of a mis-folded protein product that is not degraded, as suggested in breast carcinomas [34].

In the majority of high grade astrocytomas, specifically in grade IV glioblastomas, we observed an intense cav-1 staining at the plasma membrane (Fig. 4.1). Since the cav-1 gene maps to chromosome 7q, and that chromosome 7 gains are frequently present in glioblastomas [39–41], it cannot be excluded that the increased cav-1 expression in these subset of tumors could depend on gene amplification.

Importantly, using primary cell cultures obtained from glial tumors of different grades, we could confirm the results obtained with primary tumor specimens. As expected, cav-1 expression was significantly higher in glioblastoma cells (grade IV) than in grade III astrocytoma cells, as assessed by flow cytometry [37]. In addition, confocal microscopic studies confirmed that the pattern of cav-1 distribution varies among the different tumor types. In glioblastoma-derived cells, cav-1 is mainly located near the cell surface and its distribution participates in plasmalemma unfolding.

In recent years, gene expression profiling has identified molecular subclasses of high-grade gliomas, which display significant differences in clinical behavior [42, 43]. Specifically, recurrent gliomas with a poor prognosis showed enhanced angiogenesis as well as a cell pattern that evolved toward a mesenchymal phenotype. Genes upregulated in mesenchymal-like gliomas included, among others, a classical mesenchymal marker such as vimentin, angiogenetic markers such as VEGF and its receptors, and the endothelial marker PECAM. A previous study also demonstrated, by integrated array-comparative genomic hybridization and expression array profiles, that the cav-1 gene was among the clustered genes overexpressed in the glioblastoma subpopulation with poorer survival [44]. Further studies will be required to define if cav-1 could be considered as one of the proteins involved in the "mesenchymal transition" of brain tumors.

To date, an interesting key for interpreting the role of cav-1 in gliomas comes from some studies searching for overexpressed molecules involved in cell adhesion processes and invasiveness. In 2000, using DNA and tissue microarrays, Sallinen et al. [45] showed that the cav-1 gene was 5.2-fold increased in glioblastoma when compared with normal brain. More recently, cav-1 has been shown to regulate growth, clonogenicity, and trans-migration of glioblastoma cells, and $\alpha5\beta1$ integrin was identified as the principal mediator of cav-1 effects [46]. This coupling between cav-1 and $\alpha5\beta1$ could assume relevant usefulness for therapeutic strategies, since gliomas characterized by low cav-1/high $\alpha5\beta1$ levels are highly proliferative and infiltrative but highly responsive to $\alpha5\beta1$ integrin antagonists, whereas high cav-1/ low $\alpha5\beta1$ levels could indicate a reduced response to the drug. These data indicate that the cav-1/$\alpha5\beta1$ integrin partnership could be crucial in understanding the biology of gliomas [46].

Cav-1 in Oligodendroglial Tumors: A Different Clue?

In our first series of glial tumors studied, we reported that, as opposed to astrocytic-derived tumors (which were in their totality expressing cav-1, although with variable percentage of positive cells, staining intensity and pattern), cav-1 was mainly absent in oligendroglial tumors [37] (Fig. 4.2). In fact, of the 22 pure oligodendrogliomas tested, all those of grade II were cav-1 negative and only a minority (30%) of the grade III anaplastic tumors showed cav-1 immunoreactivity. Such data support our hypothesis of a reliable role for cav-1 as a diagnostic tool in distinguishing between low grade tumors of astrocytic *vs* oligodendroglial origin. Following this observation, we were curious to determine whether the subpopulation of cav-1 positive oligodendroglial tumors had different behavior characteristics compared with its cav-1 negative counterpart. Therefore, we studied a larger cohort of 87 pure and mixed oligodendroglial tumors and first looked for a correlation between cav-1 expression and the presence of a 1p/19q deletion, which to date represents a major prognostic/predictive factor in these tumors [47]. In fact, genetic alterations are nowadays considered extremely important in oligodendroglial tumors. For instance, it was previously reported that isolated 1p or codeletion of 1p/19q defines a subgroup of tumors, either grade II or III, with longer disease-free and overall survival [48–50]. However, although two controlled studies reported that 1p/19q loss has a definite prognostic importance, regardless of the treatment received (radiotherapy or radiotherapy + chemotherapy), Weller et al. [51] conversely suggested that the presence of a 1p/19q deletion was not a prognostic factor in patients that did not receive radio- or chemotherapy, but rather being exclusively a predictive factor for a better response to therapy [52, 53]. In addition, tumors carrying the 1p/19q deletion have a better response to first line therapy but not to salvage treatment [54]. Taken together, these conflicting results suggested the need for a novel and trustworthy prognostic marker in oligodendroglial tumors and encouraged us to search not only for a relationship between cav-1 expression and 1p/19q status but also for a possible prognostic role of cav-1 itself in these tumors. First, we confirmed and extended our previous data on cav-1 expression in gliomas and reported that cav-1 was expressed to a higher extent in mixed oligoastrocytomas (35%) compared with pure oligodendrogliomas (9%), probably because of their astroglial component. In addition, cav-1 appeared to be expressed in the majority of glioblastomas with oligodendroglial component (71%) [47]. Importantly, we provided evidences of an inverse correlation between cav-1 expression and 1p/19q status in oligodendroglial tumors. In our study, the presence of 1p/19q codeletion and cav-1 expression were mutually exclusive [47]. Furthermore, cav-1 expression negatively modulated the prognostic relevance of the 1p/19q status. In fact, 2 out of 3 cav-1 positive cases with a 1p deletion died shortly. Despite the small number of patients, the poor outcome of these cav-1 positive cases carrying a single deletion may suggest that cav-1 expression can counterbalance the favorable impact of chromosome loss [49]. However, in another study looking at the possible relationship between cav-1 expression and 1p/19q codeletion in oligodendroglial tumors, Barresi et al. [38] did not find any significant correlation between cav-1 expression and the 1p/19q deletion. This could be due to the limited number of tumors with oligodendroglial component studied in their cohort (28 cases). Moreover, only 18 of 28 cases were tested for the 1p/19q status and only 2 of these did not show deletions.

In our study, in parallel with an inverse correlation between cav-1 expression and 1p/19q codeletion in glial tumors with oligodendroglial component, we observed, by univariate analysis, that cav-1 positivity was significantly associated with a shorter survival, both in the totality of patients studied (including low and high grade tumors) and in the subgroup of high grade tumors alone. Moreover, by multivariate analysis, cav-1 expression was the unique factor retaining independent prognostic significance in this subgroup of high grade, pure or mixed, oligodendroglial tumors [47].

These results introduced the challenging idea of using immunohistochemical analysis of cav-1 expression as a reliable prognostic marker for oligodendroglial tumors. This would provide an interesting advantage over molecular analysis pre-screening (either FISH or other genetic approaches) as it is definitely an easier and cheaper technical procedure, with a favorable cost-benefit balance and a wider distribution in pathology laboratories.

Cav-1 Expression in Glioma Vasculature

The expression of cav-1 in brain microvessels has been reported by various authors [17, 19, 55, 56], mainly in relation to its role in the formation of the blood–brain barrier. Regina et al. [57] studied the regulation of cav-1 expression in the brain tumoral vasculature, and observed a down-regulation of cav-1 expression in endothelial cells isolated from brain tumors. However, since the decrease of total cav-1 was higher than the decrease of its phosphorylated counterpart (pcav-1), the ratio of pcav-1/cav-1 was highly increased in endothelial cells obtained from brain tumors when compared with normal brains. In addition, ERK1/2 phosphorylation was observed in endothelial cells obtained from brain tumors compared to normal brains. Since previous evidences demonstrated a negative regulation of ERK signaling by cav-1 [24, 58, 59], these data could be relevant in the modulation of mitogenic cascades. In addition, in another study, pcav-1 has been described to localize at the cell focal adhesion regions, major sites of tyrosine kinase signaling [60]. Despite these intriguing results, the exact role of cav-1 phosphorylation in brain tumor endothelial cells and angiogenic processes still needs to be determined.

Finally, irradiation of brain tumor endothelial cells increases cav-1 expression, restoring the levels to those detected in normal brains [57]. This result might indicate that irradiation promotes a "return" of the brain tumor vasculature to a normal status, possibly through maturation of the capillary network, which is in contrast to the angiogenic role ascribed to cav-1 phosphorylation under neoplastic condition.

The Cav-1 "Molecular Interface": Are There Cav-1 Partners that Could Bear Therapeutic Value in Brain Tumors?

It has been previously reported that cav-1 effects are mainly dependent on its coupling with various heterogeneous partner molecules [3, 4, 61]. Among these partners, EGFR deserves attention since its overexpression and its vIII variant are present in about 50% of high grade gliomas [62–65].

Moreover, EGFR expression significantly correlates with poor prognosis in intracranial ependymomas [66]. Since EGFR has been reported to be constitutively associated with cav-1 in lung carcinoma cells [67], we decided to investigate their coexpression in a series of adult supratentorial ependymomas. Interestingly, we demonstrated that cav-1 and EGFR colocalized in neoplastic cells and that their coexpression identified a subset of tumors with rapid unfavorable outcome. Interestingly, cav-1 but not EGFR expression was able to predict poor overall survival in the subset of grade II tumors, which usually represent a prognostically "gray" area [68]. In addition, recent data identified cav-1 as a marker of sensitivity to the tyrosine kinase (TKI) inhibitor dasatinib in solid tumor cell lines, which display a phenotype characterized by a mesenchymal transition [69]. This result strengthens the evidence of a functional involvement of cav-1 in the Scr family kinase (SKF)-pathway, which is required for EGFR-initiated mitogenesis [69, 70], and could thus bear biological and clinical relevance in EGFR-positive tumors of glial/ependymal origin.

Last but not least, the cav-1-dependent EGFR internalization/trafficking has been reported to be modulated by oxidative stress in lung carcinoma cells *in vitro* [67]. This process was suggested to occur via the hyper-phosphorylation of cav-1, which subsequently promoted the transport of EGFR to a perinuclear location, where it is protected from degradation and consequently remained active. Similarly, radiation-induced cav-1-dependent internalization was associated with nuclear EGFR transport and triggered by Src kinase activation [71]. Although these data were obtained in human lung carcinoma and squamous carcinoma cell lines, the common use of brain irradiation following surgery for gliomas forces us to reconsider whether cav-1 could eventually be useful in understanding the controversial mechanisms of glioma radio-resistance, which involves an heterogeneous group of molecules [72], including EGFRvIII [73, 74].

Final Considerations

The role of cav-1 in brain tumors is still extremely uncertain and is worth being elucidated in further studies. Molecular, functional, and clinical approaches can all concur in identifying the involvement of cav-1 and cav-1-associated proteins in the biology of brain tumors. Hopefully, these results could soon lead to new prognostic and therapeutic perspectives for these neoplasms, which still represent a major medical challenge.

References

1. Liu P, Rudick M, Anderson RG (2002) Multiple functions of caveolin-1. J Biol Chem 277:41295–41298
2. Shaul PW, Anderson RG (1998) Role of plasmalemmal caveolae in signal transduction. Am J Physiol 275:L843–L851
3. Burgermeister E, Liscovitch M, Rocken C et al (2008) Caveats of caveolin-1 in cancer progression. Cancer Lett 268:187–201
4. Goetz JG, Lajoie P, Wiseman SM et al (2008) Caveolin-1 in tumor progression: the good, the bad and the ugly. Cancer Metastasis Rev 27:715–735

5. Lisanti MP, Scherer PE, Tang Z et al (1994) Caveolae, caveolin and caveolin-rich membrane domains: a signalling hypothesis. Trends Cell Biol 4:231–235
6. Ando T, Ishiguro H, Kimura M et al (2007) The overexpression of caveolin-1 and caveolin-2 correlates with a poor prognosis and tumor progression in esophageal squamous cell carcinoma. Oncol Rep 18:601–609
7. Bender FC, Reymond MA, Bron C et al (2000) Caveolin-1 levels are down-regulated in human colon tumors, and ectopic expression of caveolin-1 in colon carcinoma cell lines reduces cell tumorigenicity. Cancer Res 60:5870–5878
8. Campbell L, Gumbleton M, Griffiths DF (2003) Caveolin-1 overexpression predicts poor disease-free survival of patients with clinically confined renal cell carcinoma. Br J Cancer 89:1909–1913
9. Karam JA, Lotan Y, Roehrborn CG et al (2007) Caveolin-1 overexpression is associated with aggressive prostate cancer recurrence. Prostate 67:614–622
10. Lee SW, Reimer CL, Oh P et al (1998) Tumor cell growth inhibition by caveolin re-expression in human breast cancer cells. Oncogene 16:1391–1397
11. Phuoc NB, Ehara H, Gotoh T et al (2007) Immunohistochemical analysis with multiple antibodies in search of prognostic markers for clear cell renal cell carcinoma. Urology 69:843–848
12. Wiechen K, Diatchenko L, Agoulnik A et al (2001) Caveolin-1 is down-regulated in human ovarian carcinoma and acts as a candidate tumor suppressor gene. Am J Pathol 159:1635–1643
13. Wiechen K, Sers C, Agoulnik A et al (2001) Down-regulation of caveolin-1, a candidate tumor suppressor gene, in sarcomas. Am J Pathol 158:833–839
14. Witkiewicz AK, Casimiro MC, Dasgupta A et al (2009) Towards a new "stromal-based" classification system for human breast cancer prognosis and therapy. Cell Cycle 8:1654–1658
15. Witkiewicz AK, Dasgupta A, Sotgia F et al (2009) An absence of stromal caveolin-1 expression predicts early tumor recurrence and poor clinical outcome in human breast cancers. Am J Pathol 174:2023–2034
16. Cameron PL, Ruffin JW, Bollag R et al (1997) Identification of caveolin and caveolin-related proteins in the brain. J Neurosci 17:9520–9535
17. Ikezu T, Ueda H, Trapp BD et al (1998) Affinity-purification and characterization of caveolins from the brain: differential expression of caveolin-1, -2, and -3 in brain endothelial and astroglial cell types. Brain Res 804:177–192
18. Megias L, Guerri C, Fornas E et al (2000) Endocytosis and transcytosis in growing astrocytes in primary culture. Possible implications in neural development. Int J Dev Biol 44:209–221
19. Virgintino D, Robertson D, Errede M et al (2002) Expression of caveolin-1 in human brain microvessels. Neuroscience 115:145–152
20. Bagnoli M, Tomassetti A, Figini M et al (2000) Downmodulation of caveolin-1 expression in human ovarian carcinoma is directly related to alpha-folate receptor overexpression. Oncogene 19:4754–4763
21. Koleske AJ, Baltimore D, Lisanti MP (1995) Reduction of caveolin and caveolae in oncogenically transformed cells. Proc Natl Acad Sci USA 92:1381–1385
22. Racine C, Belanger M, Hirabayashi H et al (1999) Reduction of caveolin 1 gene expression in lung carcinoma cell lines. Biochem Biophys Res Commun 255:580–586
23. Suzuki T, Suzuki Y, Hanada K et al (1998) Reduction of caveolin-1 expression in tumorigenic human cell hybrids. J Biochem 124:383–388
24. Engelman JA, Zhang XL, Lisanti MP (1998) Genes encoding human caveolin-1 and -2 are co-localized to the D7S522 locus (7q31.1), a known fragile site (FRA7G) that is frequently deleted in human cancers. FEBS Lett 436:403–410
25. Fra AM, Mastroianni N, Mancini M et al (1999) Human caveolin-1 and caveolin-2 are closely linked genes colocalized with WI-5336 in a region of 7q31 frequently deleted in tumors. Genomics 56:355–356
26. Hurlstone AF, Reid G, Reeves JR et al (1999) Analysis of the CAVEOLIN-1 gene at human chromosome 7q31.1 in primary tumours and tumour-derived cell lines. Oncogene 18:1881–1890
27. Lin JC, Scherer SW, Tougas L et al (1996) Detailed deletion mapping with a refined physical map of 7q31 localizes a putative tumor suppressor gene for breast cancer in the region of MET. Oncogene 13:2001–2008

28. Silva WI, Maldonado HM, Lisanti MP et al (1999) Identification of caveolae and caveolin in C6 glioma cells. Int J Dev Neurosci 17:705–714
29. Silva WI, Maldonado HM, Velazquez G et al (2005) Caveolin isoform expression during differentiation of C6 glioma cells. Int J Dev Neurosci 23:599–612
30. Cameron PL, Liu C, Smart DK et al (2002) Caveolin-1 expression is maintained in rat and human astroglioma cell lines. Glia 37:275–290
31. Hayashi K, Matsuda S, Machida K et al (2001) Invasion activating caveolin-1 mutation in human scirrhous breast cancers. Cancer Res 61:2361–2364
32. Bonuccelli G, Casimiro MC, Sotgia F et al (2009) Caveolin-1 (P132L), a common breast cancer mutation, confers mammary cell invasiveness and defines a novel stem cell/metastasis-associated gene signature. Am J Pathol 174:1650–1662
33. Lee H, Park DS, Razani B et al (2002) Caveolin-1 mutations (P132L and null) and the pathogenesis of breast cancer: caveolin-1 (P132L) behaves in a dominant-negative manner and caveolin-1 (-/-) null mice show mammary epithelial cell hyperplasia. Am J Pathol 161:357–369
34. Mercier I, Bryant KG, Sotgia F et al (2009) Using Caveolin-1 epithelial immunostaining patterns to stratify human breast cancer patients and predict the Caveolin-1 (P132L) mutation. Cell Cycle 8:1396–1401
35. Forget MA, Desrosiers RR, Del M et al (2002) The expression of rho proteins decreases with human brain tumor progression: potential tumor markers. Clin Exp Metastasis 19:9–15
36. Abulrob A, Giuseppin S, Andrade MF et al (2004) Interactions of EGFR and caveolin-1 in human glioblastoma cells: evidence that tyrosine phosphorylation regulates EGFR association with caveolae. Oncogene 23:6967–6979
37. Cassoni P, Senetta R, Castellano I et al (2007) Caveolin-1 expression is variably displayed in astroglial-derived tumors and absent in oligodendrogliomas: concrete premises for a new reliable diagnostic marker in gliomas. Am J Surg Pathol 31:760–769
38. Barresi V, Buttarelli FR, Vitarelli EE et al (2009) Caveolin-1 expression in diffuse gliomas: correlation with the proliferation index, epidermal growth factor receptor, p53, and 1p/19q status. Hum Pathol 40:1738–1746
39. Ichimura K, Ohgaki H, Kleihues P et al (2004) Molecular pathogenesis of astrocytic tumours. J Neurooncol 70:137–160
40. Misra A, Pellarin M, Nigro J et al (2005) Array comparative genomic hybridization identifies genetic subgroups in grade 4 human astrocytoma. Clin Cancer Res 11:2907–2918
41. Wiltshire RN, Herndon JE 2nd, Lloyd A et al (2004) Comparative genomic hybridization analysis of astrocytomas: prognostic and diagnostic implications. J Mol Diagn 6:166–179
42. Nigro JM, Misra A, Zhang L et al (2005) Integrated array-comparative genomic hybridization and expression array profiles identify clinically relevant molecular subtypes of glioblastoma. Cancer Res 65:1678–1686
43. Phillips HS, Kharbanda S, Chen R et al (2006) Molecular subclasses of high-grade glioma predict prognosis, delineate a pattern of disease progression, and resemble stages in neurogenesis. Cancer Cell 9:157–173
44. Godard S, Getz G, Delorenzi M et al (2003) Classification of human astrocytic gliomas on the basis of gene expression: a correlated group of genes with angiogenic activity emerges as a strong predictor of subtypes. Cancer Res 63:6613–6625
45. Sallinen SL, Sallinen PK, Haapasalo HK et al (2000) Identification of differentially expressed genes in human gliomas by DNA microarray and tissue chip techniques. Cancer Res 60:6617–6622
46. Martin S, Cosset EC, Terrand J et al (2009) Caveolin-1 regulates glioblastoma aggressiveness through the control of alpha(5)beta(1) integrin expression and modulates glioblastoma responsiveness to SJ749, an alpha(5)beta(1) integrin antagonist. Biochim Biophys Acta 1793:354–367
47. Senetta R, Trevisan E, Ruda R et al (2009) Caveolin 1 expression independently predicts shorter survival in oligodendrogliomas. J Neuropathol Exp Neurol 68:425–431
48. Iwamoto FM, Nicolardi L, Demopoulos A et al (2008) Clinical relevance of 1p and 19q deletion for patients with WHO grade 2 and 3 gliomas. J Neurooncol 88:293–298

49. Kujas M, Lejeune J, Benouaich-Amiel A et al (2005) Chromosome 1p loss: a favorable prognostic factor in low-grade gliomas. Ann Neurol 58:322–326
50. Mariani L, Deiana G, Vassella E et al (2006) Loss of heterozygosity 1p36 and 19q13 is a prognostic factor for overall survival in patients with diffuse WHO grade 2 gliomas treated without chemotherapy. J Clin Oncol 24:4758–4763
51. Weller M, Berger H, Hartmann C et al (2007) Combined 1p/19q loss in oligodendroglial tumors: predictive or prognostic biomarker? Clin Cancer Res 13:6933–6937
52. Cairncross G, Berkey B, Shaw E et al (2006) Phase III trial of chemotherapy plus radiotherapy compared with radiotherapy alone for pure and mixed anaplastic oligodendroglioma: Intergroup Radiation Therapy Oncology Group Trial 9402. J Clin Oncol 24:2707–2714
53. van den Bent MJ, Carpentier AF, Brandes AA et al (2006) Adjuvant procarbazine, lomustine, and vincristine improves progression-free survival but not overall survival in newly diagnosed anaplastic oligodendrogliomas and oligoastrocytomas: a randomized European Organisation for Research and Treatment of Cancer phase III trial. J Clin Oncol 24:2715–2722
54. Kouwenhoven MC, Kros JM, French PJ et al (2006) 1p/19q loss within oligodendroglioma is predictive for response to first line temozolomide but not to salvage treatment. Eur J Cancer 42:2499–2503
55. Jodoin J, Demeule M, Fenart L et al (2003) P-glycoprotein in blood-brain barrier endothelial cells: interaction and oligomerization with caveolins. J Neurochem 87:1010–1023
56. Song L, Ge S, Pachter JS (2007) Caveolin-1 regulates expression of junction-associated proteins in brain microvascular endothelial cells. Blood 109:1515–1523
57. Regina A, Jodoin J, Khoueir P et al (2004) Down-regulation of caveolin-1 in glioma vasculature: modulation by radiotherapy. J Neurosci Res 75:291–299
58. Engelman JA, Wykoff CC, Yasuhara S et al (1997) Recombinant expression of caveolin-1 in oncogenically transformed cells abrogates anchorage-independent growth. J Biol Chem 272:16374–16381
59. Galbiati F, Volonte D, Engelman JA et al (1998) Targeted downregulation of caveolin-1 is sufficient to drive cell transformation and hyperactivate the p42/44 MAP kinase cascade. EMBO J 17:6633–6648
60. Brown G, Rixon HW, Sugrue RJ (2002) Respiratory syncytial virus assembly occurs in GM1-rich regions of the host-cell membrane and alters the cellular distribution of tyrosine phosphorylated caveolin-1. J Gen Virol 83:1841–1850
61. Williams TM, Lisanti MP (2005) Caveolin-1 in oncogenic transformation, cancer, and metastasis. Am J Physiol 288:C494–C506
62. Hurtt MR, Moossy J, Donovan-Peluso M et al (1992) Amplification of epidermal growth factor receptor gene in gliomas: histopathology and prognosis. J Neuropathol Exp Neurol 51:84–90
63. Lo HW, Cao X, Zhu H et al (2008) Constitutively activated STAT3 frequently coexpresses with epidermal growth factor receptor in high-grade gliomas and targeting STAT3 sensitizes them to Iressa and alkylators. Clin Cancer Res 14:6042–6054
64. Schlegel J, Merdes A, Stumm G et al (1994) Amplification of the epidermal-growth-factor-receptor gene correlates with different growth behaviour in human glioblastoma. Int J Cancer 56:72–77
65. Schlegel J, Stumm G, Brandle K et al (1994) Amplification and differential expression of members of the erbB-gene family in human glioblastoma. J Neurooncol 22:201–207
66. Mendrzyk F, Korshunov A, Benner A et al (2006) Identification of gains on 1q and epidermal growth factor receptor overexpression as independent prognostic markers in intracranial ependymoma. Clin Cancer Res 12:2070–2079
67. Khan EM, Heidinger JM, Levy M et al (2006) Epidermal growth factor receptor exposed to oxidative stress undergoes Src- and caveolin-1-dependent perinuclear trafficking. J Biol Chem 281:14486–14493
68. Senetta R, Miracco C, Lanzafame S et al (2011) Epidermal growth factor receptor and caveolin-1 coexpression identifies adult supratentorial ependymomas with rapid unfavourable outcomes. Neuro Oncol 13:176–183

69. Huang F, Reeves K, Han X et al (2007) Identification of candidate molecular markers predicting sensitivity in solid tumors to dasatinib: rationale for patient selection. Cancer Res 67:2226–2238
70. Thomas SM, Brugge JS (1997) Cellular functions regulated by Src family kinases. Annu Rev Cell Dev Biol 13:513–609
71. Dittmann K, Mayer C, Kehlbach R et al (2008) Radiation-induced caveolin-1 associated EGFR internalization is linked with nuclear EGFR transport and activation of DNA-PK. Mol Cancer 7:69
72. Wang J, Wakeman TP, Lathia JD et al (2010) Notch promotes radioresistance of glioma stem cells. Stem cells 28:17-28
73. Golding SE, Morgan RN, Adams BR et al (2009) Pro-survival AKT and ERK signaling from EGFR and mutant EGFRvIII enhances DNA double-strand break repair in human glioma cells. Cancer Biol Ther 8:730–738
74. Mukherjee B, McEllin B, Camacho CV et al (2009) EGFRvIII and DNA double-strand break repair: a molecular mechanism for radioresistance in glioblastoma. Cancer Res 69:4252–4259

Chapter 5
The Role of Caveolin-1 in Skin Cancer

Alessandra Carè, Isabella Parolini, Federica Felicetti,
and Massimo Sargiacomo

Introduction

Since the first description that caveolin (Cav-1) homo-oligomeric complexes are able to regulate signal transduction in caveolae [23], more knowledge on Cav-1 functions in physiological processes has been achieved. Among various multiprotein complexes present as transient cell surface signaling microdomains on the plasma membrane, Cav-1 appears as a ubiquitous adapter molecule able to affect the morphology or function of cells. In fact, Cav-1 possesses a scaffolding domain (CSD; aa 82–101), which interacts with partner proteins, thereby concentrating downstream signaling cascades into the invaginations of plasma membrane caveolae. Consequently, the physiological impact of Cav-1 in normal or pathophysiological conditions may rely on the specific molecular partners encountered. The modulation of Cav-1 expression and/or function was hypothesized to play a role in human cancer and other disease pathogenesis [24, 36]. Several studies implicate that Cav-1 fulfills a tumor-suppressor role in vitro and in vivo [34]. However, others reported increased expression of Cav-1 in the more advanced stages of cancers [11, 12]. Hence, the apparent contradictory Cav-1 behaviors could be explained by the presence of a scaffolding domain, which could account for the formation of integrated but variable functional protein multicomplexes [3]. The inhibitory actions of Cav-1 on cell growth have been demonstrated by the enhanced susceptibility of Cav-1 KO mice toward chemically-induced carcinogenesis (reviewed in [34]). Moreover, data obtained from ectopic re-expression of Cav-1 in Cav-1 KO mouse embryonic fibroblasts and various other transformed cells led to the persuasion that Cav-1 acts as a tumor suppressor. However, early results of Cav-1 deficiency in primary tumors completely contrasted with more recent data, in that Cav-1 re-acquisition associates

A. Carè • I. Parolini • F. Felicetti • M. Sargiacomo (✉)
Department of Hematology, Oncology and Molecular Medicine, Istituto Superiore di Sanità,
Viale Regina Elena, 299-00161 Rome, Italy
e-mail: massimo.sargiacomo@iss.it

I. Mercier et al. (eds.), *Caveolins in Cancer Pathogenesis, Prevention and Therapy*,
Current Cancer Research, DOI 10.1007/978-1-4614-1001-0_5,
© Springer Science+Business Media, LLC 2012

with advanced cancer stages as seen in colon, breast, prostate, bladder, esophagus, and thyroid tumors (reviewed in [3]). Thus, the proposed antithetic roles of Cav-1 are in agreement with its variable molecular arrangements in a given cellular or animal model that is consistent with the definition of scaffold proteins.

A possible example of Cav-1 inhibitory effect on tumor progression involves Cav-1 and the regulation of integrin alpha /Fyn /Shc /Ras /ERK pathway for an anchorage-dependent cell growth [33]. In contrast, high levels of intracellular Cav-1 expression have been consistently associated with metastatic progression of human prostate cancer and other malignancies, including lung, renal, and esophageal squamous cell cancers [3]. Interestingly, discrepancies in Cav-1 expression have also emerged within melanoma cancer cell lines. This issue will be the focus of this chapter dedicated to Cav-1 and skin cancer.

Cav-1 in Skin Cancer

Skin cancer is the most common form of neoplasia in the United States. The two most common, but likely highly curable types, are basal cell cancer and squamous cell carcinomas. Conversely, melanoma is rare, but very aggressive. In the last decades, its incidence is steadily increasing in most countries, while not paralleled by the development of new therapeutic agents with a significant impact on survival. At present, early detected melanomas can be cured by surgical excision, while more advanced stages are difficult to control. Once melanomas metastasize, the median 5-year survival rate is less than 5% [18]. At present, few data exist on Cav-1 expression and function in non-melanoma skin cancers. A microarray-based gene profiling showed increased Cav-1 expression in human basal cell carcinomas (BCC) as compared to normal skin, suggesting that it may play a dynamic role in controlling the slow progression of these tumors through both decreased cellular motility and tumor promotion [25]. We will give a first appraisal of Cav-1 expression in skin cancer based quite exclusively on recent data obtained from melanoma studies. The original purpose of this chapter is to bring attention to the role of Cav-1-containing vesicles (exosomes) secreted by melanoma cancer cells. Exosomes are relatively well-characterized entities secreted by diverse cells through a specific intracellular pathway involving multivesicular bodies (MVB) or endosomal-related regions of the plasma membrane implicated in intercellular transfer of specific signaling proteins. Recent studies have reported that secreted exosomes contain a subset of cellular proteins, mRNAs, and microRNAs (miRNAs), which can be transferred to and translated within recipient cells [32]. We suggest that exosomal secretion may be a key mode of communication among human melanoma cells analogous to prosta-somes in prostate cancer [15], and that this secretion is sensitive to microenviron-mental pH [22]. Finally, we will discuss the presence of detectable quantity of Cav-1-containing exosomes in the plasma of metastatic patients and in culture media from human melanoma cells [9, 16].

Cav-1 Is Down or Upregulated in Melanoma Cells

Focusing on the role of Cav-1 in malignant melanoma emerges once again as a complex picture. The overall data on Cav-1 show that it possesses dual functions within the same cancer, either as a pro- or anti-metastatic protein.

Historically, the murine B16 melanoma cell system, especially through its subclone B16F, was chosen as a model for studying tumor cell and host properties in association with metastases [21]. More recently, B16F cells were utilized to explore the function of Cav-1 in melanoma development and dissemination [31]. Since this work is the last of a list of papers based on B16 melanoma cell lines, studies on the role of the *Cav-1* gene on metastasis formation in this system deserve a closer examination.

The low Cav-1 expressing B16F10 cells, a B16-derived murine melanoma cell line, were selected for their uniqueness to colonize lung and, as an experimental system, to assess the effects of Cav-1 re-introduction in these tumor cells [31]. Specifically, Trimmer and coworkers showed that Cav-1 overexpression induces B16F10 cell proliferation by increasing the percentage of cells in the S and G_2/M phases, but inhibits the migratory abilities of B16F10 cells in vitro and in vivo. Accordingly, Cav-1 enforced expression appears able to repress Src and FAK activities following integrin engagement.

It has to be noted that since the earliest studies on rafts and caveolae in B16 cells, it came out a peculiarity regarding these highly selected cells [35]. In fact, these cells demonstrated a complete separation between ganglioside sphingolipid (GSL)-microdomains and caveolae, based on clear cut differences in lipid composition and plasma membrane location. Accordingly, only GM3-GSL rafts isolated from B16 cells contained transducer molecules (c-Src, Rho, Ras, FAK), integrin receptors and tyrosine kinase-linked growth factor receptors. Thus in B16 cells, GSL-enriched microdomains are structurally and functionally different from caveolae and autonomously capable of causing cell adhesion as well as signal transduction (glycosignaling domain). Further concerns about this cell line might come from contradictory effects generated by gangliosides themselves in cell signaling [13]. Thus, we believe that B16 cells represent a very special tumor system that seems independent of Cav-1 and mostly rely on GM3 ganglioside. Thus, the reversal effects described [31] by the re-expression of Cav-1 in B16 cells in terms of signaling and lung colonization might not be completely specific and need to be better clarified at a molecular level to examine Cav-1-forming protein complexes.

The histological evidences provided by Trimmer et al. showing the lack of Cav-1 in a panel of human metastatic melanoma tissues renders this data interesting and unique among the published literature. Carefully searching on this topic, we found a study on gastric carcinoma (GC) as an interesting parallel of the aforementioned melanoma tissue results, in that immunohistological experiments confirmed how cells in advanced tumor stage are mostly devoid of Cav-1 [4]. However, in the same study, further histological observations revealed a number of Cav-1-positive metastatic cell lines directly derived from those tissues. In particular, Cav-1 expression was higher among cells originating from distal metastases [4].

Table 5.1 Expression of endogenous and exosome-associated Cav-1 in primary and metastatic melanoma cell lines

Cell line	Type	Cellular Cav-1	Exosome-associated Cav-1
WM983A	Primary tumor VGP	–	–
Me1007	Primary tumor VGP	–/+	–
A375	Metastatic melanoma	++	++
Me665/1	Lymph node metastasis	++++	++++
Me1811	Lymph node metastasis	+++	++

VGP: vertical growth phase

In contrast to data showing the potential tumor-suppressor activities of Cav-1, numerous studies have also documented the overexpression of Cav-1 in malignant tissues [27, 30, 34], including human melanoma [9].

Our investigations on a panel of melanomas showed Cav-1 expression in all the analyzed cell lines (Table 5.1). The exception was a primary vertical melanoma cell line characterized by the lack of Cav-1, and then utilized as a recipient for Cav-1 gene transduction to address a series of functional studies. The retrovirally driven re-expression of Cav-1 in this melanoma cell line effectively increased cell growth, anchorage-independence, as well as migration and invasion capabilities. Conversely, Cav-1 silencing in metastatic Cav-1-positive melanoma cell lines clearly reduced their proliferative rates as well as their tumorigenicity. These functional data were supported by a Cav-1-dependent upregulation of metalloproteases, MMP-2 and MMP-9, known to directly correlate with a more invasive phenotype in tumor cells [9].

In addition, Cav-1 expression was found to positively associate with melanoma malignancy, being low in primary melanomas and highly expressed in cell lines derived from lymph node metastases (Table 5.1). In the same study, we detected a secreted exosome-associated fraction of Cav-1 in melanoma conditioned media (see Table 5.1), directly proportional to endogenous Cav-1 expression. Interestingly, this data was in line with another study on prostate cancer where serum levels of Cav-1 were proposed as diagnostic and prognostic markers [28].

Accordingly, Cav-1 has been identified as a serum marker that is significantly expressed in melanoma patients when compared with healthy controls [16]. These results (further discussed below) showed a direct correlation between plasma Cav-1 levels and tumor stage in patients. Thus confirming its pro-neoplastic role in human melanoma.

In our experiments, Cav-1 expression in human melanoma-derived cell lines was unquestionably associated with its tumor-promoting function, while Cav-1 immunodetection on the corresponding melanoma tissues is still lacking. However, studies on GC demonstrated a stage-dependent Cav-1 expression with a biphasic differential function in original tissue and derived cell lines [4], namely low in tissue and high in cell lines. In GC, Cav-1 appears as a survival factor whose overexpression is required for cancer dissemination. Altogether, these findings address a complex and possible dual behavior of Cav-1. In this view, another important clue is given by the tissue context itself that must confer additional and crucial information on the role of Cav-1, as suggested by the significant inverse correlation between stromal and epithelial Cav-1 levels observed in prostate cancer [7].

Phosphorylated Cav-1 Is Implicated in Melanoma Progression

The dual role of Cav-1 might be explained by post-translational modifications causing changes in the conformation and subcellular localization of Cav-1, as well as its association with different partner molecules. A well-described modification consists in the Src-dependent phosphorylation at tyrosine-14 (Y14) of the N-terminal domain of Cav-1 (ph-Cav-1), which induces proliferation and anchorage-independent growth via the Ras/Raf/Erk cascade. In addition, the phosphorylation on tyrosine 14 removes the ability of the CSD to inhibit the activity of growth factor receptor tyrosine kinases (e.g., neu/ErbB2/Her2) [34]. Cav-1 can be phosphorylated by oncogenic transformation and upon various stimuli (IGF-I, EGF, insulin) or different stress conditions. Moreover, Y14-phosphorylation has been associated with Cav-1 translocation and clustering with integrins as part of focal adhesions [6], suggestive of a role in cell adhesion, migration, and invasion. A balance between unphosphorylated and ph-Cav-1 might influence its tumor-suppressing or -promoting functional roles.

The role of the phosphorylation status of Cav-1 was demonstrated in melanoma where we transfected the wild-type Cav-1 and a non-phosphorylatable mutant (Cav-1-Y14A) into a Cav-1-negative primary melanoma cell line [9]. The role of Cav-1 on the different levels of malignancy was then analyzed through in vitro migration assays. The effects observed in Cav-1-expressing cells were strictly related to its phosphorylation levels as demonstrated by the abrogation of tumorigenicity in the presence of the Cav-1-Y14A non-phosphorylatable mutant. The functional involvement of ph-Cav-1 was also confirmed by treatment with the Src-family kinase inhibitor PP1, which strongly reduced the chemotactic ability of melanoma cells [9].

Cav-1-Containing Exosomes Are Secreted by Melanoma Cells

Exosomes are biological nanoparticles ranging between 30 and 100 nm in size, originating from the inward budding of MVBs, a component of the endocytic pathway, and subsequent release into the surrounding extracellular space through fusion with the cellular plasma membrane. In normal cell systems, exosomes are constitutively secreted by dendritic cells and macrophages, or after cell surface receptor activation by reticulocytes, T cells, mastocytes, and B cells [29]. Tumor cells naturally release abundant exosomes in the extracellular space to support tumor cell survival, growth, tissue invasion and metastasis [2]. Accordingly, exosomes have been found in the serum of patients with tumors, with increased amounts in patients with advanced cancers.

Recent studies highlighted the theory that exosomes may represent a novel way of intercellular communication alternative to soluble protein–receptor interactions. In fact exosomes are endowed of different molecules (proteins, soluble factors, RNAs, and miRNAs) specific to the producing cells, which are capable to confer new properties to a recipient cell. This appears to be of great importance for the pathogenesis of tumors.

EXOSOME MEDIATED TRANSFER

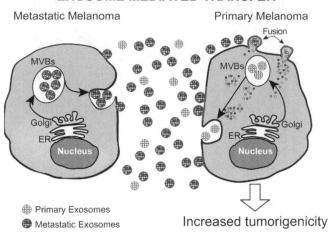

Fig. 5.1 Schematic representation of exosome-mediated cell to cell communication. Exosomes, abundantly released by metastatic melanoma cells, are taken up through a fusion mechanism by primary melanoma recipients. The induction of a more malignant phenotype is associated with the transfer of metastases-related molecules, including Cav-1/Ph-Cav-1, MMP-9 and miR-221/-222

Because of their ability to circulate and transport a broad spectrum of proteins deriving from different compartments of the producing cell, exosomes can be considered important molecule reservoirs, whose decipherment might shed light on the mechanisms underlying tumor progression. Thus, for the first time in our laboratory, the molecular analysis of human melanoma-secreted exosomes was used to elucidate the aforementioned controversial role of Cav-1 in melanoma progression. We clearly observed that metastatic melanoma cells release exosomes in the extracellular space in higher proportion than primary melanoma [9], and that these vesicles express higher amounts of Cav-1, and ph-Cav-1. More importantly, Cav-1-bearing exosomes are capable of a horizontal transfer from metastatic to less aggressive melanomas, in turn promoting their invasive activity. Representative markers were utilized to confirm the effective exosomal transfer of molecules associated with the more aggressive phenotype into the primary melanoma cell membranes [9]. Among them, MMP-9 detected in purified exosomes from human metastatic cell lines could also be found in primary cells after fusion with metastatic-derived exosomes. These results confirmed the transport of molecules from cell to cell as a function of tumor aggressiveness and progression. Accordingly, functional studies showed an increase in the tumorigenic properties of a primary melanoma cell line following the up-take of metastatic-secreted vesicles [9] (see Fig. 5.1).

Interestingly, among these relevant molecules, we also found miRNAs, which are regulatory RNAs that act as post-transcriptional repressors by binding the 3' untranslated region of target genes. In the last few years, their abnormal expression and functional role in cancer have been unmistakably demonstrated. In particular, we reported miR-221 and miR-222 abnormal expressions in melanoma, with increasing expression throughout the stepwise transformation process from normal melanocytes to metastases. The enhanced expression of miR-221/222 activates at least two important pathways governing cell proliferation and melanogenesis through the regulation of p27 Kip1 and the c-KIT receptor, respectively [8].

Recently, circulating miRNas have also been detected in both plasma and serum of healthy and diseased subjects [14]. Specifically, extracellular miRNAs have been found either as free molecules or protected inside microvesicles/exosomes. Our ongoing studies show that secretory miRNAs in melanoma exosomes can be transferred and exert their functions in recipient cells, indicating that at least part of the intercellular communication between cancer cells and their surrounding microenvironment could involve these regulatory RNAs. In agreement with miR-221 and -222 oncogenic functions, exosomes recovered from metastatic melanoma cell lines express very high levels of these two miRNAs, further supporting their role in cancer dissemination (our unpublished results).

Melanoma Exosomes Are Highly Released in Acidic Microenvironment and in Patients' Plasma

Among the recognized and well-described exosome biological functions, several studies indicated exosomes as instruments used by cancer cells to prepare distal sites for metastatic dissemination. A good example of this is given by glioma exosomes bearing an oncogenic EGF receptor variant (EGFRvIII), which once released from normal endothelial cells can trigger a cascade pathway, leading to increased tumorigenic properties of target cells [1]. Parallel studies also reported a dramatic action of melanoma exosomes on endothelial regulation, as evidenced by spheroid growth and the formation of early vasculature precursor [10].

Studies on the molecular mechanisms of exosomes trafficking have been lacking, and it is only recently that several hypotheses have emerged either in normal or tumor cells. It has been proposed that the interaction of exosomes with recipient cells may occur through lipids [19] or ligand-receptor bindings [26]. Alternatively, exosomes may enter through endocytic compartments mediated by various receptors and by fusion of vesicles with internal endosomal membranes [20]. In a human melanoma cell system, our recent study reported that exosome internalization could take place through a membrane fusion mechanism, by using a fusion assay based on R18 lipid probe dequenching [22], previously used in viral fusion tests. This methodology, based on an exosome membrane labeling with the lipophilic probe octadecyl rhodamine B chloride (R18), allowed to efficiently and rapidly follow the uptake of exosomes in target cells. This was observed through fluorescence dequenching kinetic curves, which revealed an exosome/cell membrane fusion mechanism [22].

Some features of the tumor microenvironment may represent key factors in the regulation of exosome trafficking within the neoplastic mass. In particular, the tumor microenvironment is acidic, and it is known that acidity is involved in the regulation of some vesicle-mediated malignant cell functions, such as cannibalism and drug-resistance [5, 17]. As opposed to normal cells, malignant melanomas survive in an acidic microenvironment due to hyperfunctional proton pumps that do not allow acidification of the cytosol [17]. Thus, by using different pH experimental conditions, it was described that melanoma exosome trafficking varies as a function of microenvironmental pH. Indeed, low pH induces abundant exosome release and uptake through a membrane fusion mechanism [22]. This data was supported by membrane biophysical analyses, such as fluidity and lipid composition, which indicated a high rigidity and sphingomyelin (SM)/ganglioside GM3(GM3) contents in exosomes released at low pH [22]. GM3 is a recognized marker of highly ordered sphingolipid/ cholesterol plasma membrane microdomains, known as "lipid rafts." Sphingolipids play a key role in viral fusion with cell membranes by affecting protein binding as well as membrane physicochemical and mechanical properties. Hence, it seems conceivable that high SM+GM3 contents in the acidic exosomes positively affect their fusion ability. Therefore, a specific tumor microenvironment parameter such as acidity is able to influence exosome release. In turn, those exosomes may condition other cells and tissues through their specific cargo delivery (including Cav-1). In this regard, Cav-1-bearing exosomes secreted from metastatic melanoma are delivered to primary melanoma more efficiently in acidic than buffered condition [22].

Furthermore, the results of our study provide the evidence that exosomes may be used as a delivery system for paracrine diffusion of tumor malignancy, in turn supporting the importance of both exosomes and tumor pH as key targets for future anti-cancer strategies. Since human tumor-derived exosomes are involved in malignant progression, their presence was evaluated in the plasma of melanoma patients as a potential tool for cancer screening and follow-up, through an ELISA-based noninvasive assay [16]. Exosomes were captured and quantified by evaluating the expression of housekeeping proteins (CD63 and Rab-5b) and Cav-1. This assay was also extended to human tumor cell culture supernatants and plasma from SCID mice engrafted with human melanoma. In both cases, exosomes levels correlated with tumor size and stage [16].

Studying the molecular signature enclosed in exosomes and disseminated in patients' plasma may enormously expand our learning of the molecular steps needed for cell transformation and tumor progression. In a not too far future, based on their extreme ability to fuse and convey signals from cell to cell, exosomes will be possibly utilized as vehicles of signature molecules able to restore a normal genetic asset.

Conclusion

So far, Cav-1 function in melanoma has not been completely elucidated because of the various diverse, but possibly reconcilable, proposed model systems. Studies conducted on human melanoma-derived cell lines have shown explicit Cav-1 propensity to uphold metastasis advancement when abundantly expressed. Interestingly, the loss of Cav-1 in cancer-associated stroma inversely correlated with its increased expression in tumor epithelial cells, thus possibly explaining not only the dual role of Cav-1 in cancer, but also the apparent discrepancy between biopsy samples and stabilized cell lines. In this view, it is also important to consider the evidence of paracrine signaling between cancer cells and the tumor micro-environment.

The finding that melanoma cancer cells secrete exosomes bearing Cav-1 gives the opportunity to take advantage of its differential expression. Cav-1-containing exosomes seem to define a stage-specific melanoma, providing the basis for its exploration as a potential biomarker for prognosis and eventually therapy in melanoma patients.

Acknowledgments We thank G. Loreto for preparation of the figures. This work was partially supported by the Italian Ministry of Health (to MS and AC) and by the Italian Association for Cancer Research to AC.

References

1. Al-Nedawi K, Meehan B, Micallef J et al (2008) Intercellular transfer of the oncogenic receptor EGFRvIII by microvesicles derived from tumour cells. Nat Cell Biol 10:619–624
2. Al-Nedawi K, Meehan B, Rak J (2009) Microvesicles: Messengers and mediators of tumor progression. Cell Cycle 8:2014–2018
3. Burgermeister E, Liscovitch M, Rocken C et al (2008) Caveats of caveolin-1 in cancer progression. Cancer Lett 268:187–201
4. Burgermeister E, Xing X, Rocken C et al (2007) Differential expression and function of caveolin-1 in human gastric cancer progression. Cancer Res 67:8519–8526
5. De Milito A, Iessi E, Logozzi M et al (2007) Proton pump inhibitors induce apoptosis of human B-cell tumors through a caspase-independent mechanism involving reactive oxygen species. Cancer Res 67:5408–5417
6. del Pozo MA, Balasubramanian N, Alderson NB et al (2005) Phospho-caveolin-1 mediates integrin-regulated membrane domain internalization. Nat Cell Biol 7:901–908
7. Di Vizio D, Morello M, Sotgia F et al (2009) An absence of stromal caveolin-1 is associated with advanced prostate cancer, metastatic disease and epithelial akt activation. Cell Cycle 8:2420–2424
8. Felicetti F, Errico MC, Bottero L et al (2008) The promyelocytic leukemia zinc finger-microRNA-221/-222 pathway controls melanoma progression through multiple oncogenic mechanisms. Cancer Res 68:2745–2754
9. Felicetti F, Parolini I, Bottero L et al (2009) Caveolin-1 tumor-promoting role in human melanoma. Int J Cancer 125:1514–1522
10. Hood JL, Pan H, Lanza GM et al (2009) Paracrine induction of endothelium by tumor exosomes. Lab Invest 89:1317–1328
11. Joo HJ, Oh DK, Kim YS et al (2004) Increased expression of caveolin-1 and microvessel density correlates with metastasis and poor prognosis in clear cell renal cell carcinoma. BJU Int 93:291–296
12. Karam JA, Lotan Y, Roehrborn G et al (2007) Caveolin-1 overexpression is associated with aggressive prostate cancer recurrence. Prostate 67:614–622
13. Kaucic K, Liu Y, Ladisch S (2006) Modulation of growth factor signaling by gangliosides: Positive or negative? Methods Enzymol 417:168–185
14. Kosaka N, Iguchi H, Ochiya T (2010) Circulating microRNA in body fluid: A new potential biomarker for cancer diagnosis and prognosis. Cancer Sci 101:2087–2092
15. Llorente A, de Marco MC, Alonso MA (2004) Caveolin-1 and MAL are located on prostasomes secreted by the prostate cancer PC-3 cell line. J Cell Sci 117:5343–5351

16. Logozzi M, De Milito A, Lugini L et al (2009) High levels of exosomes expressing CD63 and caveolin-1 in plasma of melanoma patients. PLoS One 4:e5219
17. Lugini L, Matarrese P, Tinari A et al (2006) Cannibalism of live lymphocytes by human metastatic but not primary melanoma cells. Cancer Res 66:3629–3638
18. Miller AJ, Mihm MC Jr (2006) Melanoma. N Engl J Med 355:51–65
19. Miyanishi M, Tada K, Koike M et al (2007) Identification of Tim4 as a phosphatidylserine receptor. Nature 450:435–439
20. Morelli AE, Larregina AT, Shufesky WJ et al (2004) Endocytosis, intracellular sorting, and processing of exosomes by dendritic cells. Blood 104:3257–3266
21. Nicolson GL, Brunson KW, Fidler IJ (1978) Specificity of arrest, survival, and growth of selected metastatic variant cell lines. Cancer Res 38:4105–4111
22. Parolini I, Federici C, Raggi C et al (2009) Microenvironmental pH is a key factor for exosome traffic in tumor cells. J Biol Chem 284:34211–34222
23. Sargiacomo M, Scherer PE, Tang Z et al (1995) Oligomeric structure of caveolin: Implications for caveolae membrane organization. Proc Natl Acad Sci USA 92:9407–9411
24. Satoh T, Yang G, Egawa S et al (2003) Caveolin-1 expression is a predictor of recurrence-free survival in pT2N0 prostate carcinoma diagnosed in japanese patients. Cancer 97:1225–1233
25. Savage K, Lambros MB, Robertson D et al (2007) Caveolin 1 is overexpressed and amplified in a subset of basal-like and metaplastic breast carcinomas: A morphologic, ultrastructural, immunohistochemical, and in situ hybridization analysis. Clin Cancer Res 13:90–101
26. Segura E, Guerin C, Hogg N et al (2007) CD8+ dendritic cells use LFA-1 to capture MHC-peptide complexes from exosomes in vivo. J Immunol 179:1489–1496
27. Shatz M, Liscovitch M (2008) Caveolin-1: A tumor-promoting role in human cancer. Int J Radiat Biol 84:177–189
28. Tahir SA, Frolov A, Hayes TG et al (2006) Preoperative serum caveolin-1 as a prognostic marker for recurrence in a radical prostatectomy cohort. Clin Cancer Res 12:4872–4875
29. Thery C, Ostrowski M, Segura E (2009) Membrane vesicles as conveyors of immune responses. Nat Rev Immunol 9:581–593
30. Thompson TC, Tahir SA, Li L et al (2010) The role of caveolin-1 in prostate cancer: Clinical implications. Prostate Cancer Prostatic Dis 13:6–11
31. Trimmer C, Whitaker-Menezes D, Bonuccelli G et al (2010) CAV1 inhibits metastatic potential in melanomas through suppression of the integrin/Src/FAK signaling pathway. Cancer Res 70:7489–7499
32. Valadi H, Ekstrom K, Bossios A et al (2007) Exosome-mediated transfer of mRNAs and microRNAs is a novel mechanism of genetic exchange between cells. Nat Cell Biol 9:654–659
33. Wary KK, Mariotti A, Zurzolo C , Giancotti FG (1998) A requirement for Caveolin-1 and associated kinase Fyn in integrin signalling and anchorage –dependent cell growth. Cell 94:625–634
34. Williams TM, Lisanti MP (2005) Caveolin-1 in oncogenic transformation, cancer, and metastasis. Am J Physiol Cell Physiol 288:C494–C506
35. Yamamura S, Handa K, Hakomori S (1997) A close association of GM3 with c-src and rho in GM3-enriched microdomains at the B16 melanoma cell surface membrane: A preliminary note. Biochem Biophys Res Commun 236:218–222
36. Yang G, Addai J, Wheeler TM et al (2007) Correlative evidence that prostate cancer cell-derived caveolin-1 mediates angiogenesis. Hum Pathol 38:1688–1695

Chapter 6
Caveolins in Tumor Angiogenesis

Grzegorz Sowa

Introduction: Tumor-induced Angiogenesis and Angiogenic Switch

Early tumor growth is typically restricted to 2 mm in diameter. This phase is called the avascular phase, in which no formation of new tumor-associated blood vessels is observed, and a simple diffusion of oxygen and nutrients provided by nearby blood vessels is sufficient for tumor growth. To exceed the size limit of 2 mm, tumors need to gain access to an increased supply of oxygen and nutrients. The latter can only be achieved by angiogenesis, the formation of new blood vessels from pre-existing vasculature, for example, from capillaries or venules. This transition from the avascular to the angiogenic phase of tumor growth is often referred to as the "angiogenic switch" [1, 2]. The angiogenic switch and the subsequent increase in tumor blood vessel density is the most critical mechanism, which allows tumors to overcome growth limitations due to insufficient blood supply. The tumor induces the angiogenic switch by secreting pro-angiogenic and/or by suppressing antiangiogenic factors, resulting in the induction of endothelial cell (EC) proliferation and migration, vessel sprouting, and tube formation. The angiogenic switch can be triggered by tumor cells themselves, or by stromal, and tumor-infiltrating immune cells. These cells release soluble factors, the main targets of which are endothelial and other vascular cells in the tumor microenvironment. An increase in EC proliferation, followed by migration is an early indicator of angiogenic switch. Many in vitro and in vivo assays have been developed to study the process of angiogenesis and to identify pro- and anti-angiogenic factors. EC proliferation, migration, and capillary tube formation are particularly important in vitro readouts of angiogenesis [3].

G. Sowa (✉)
Department of Medical Pharmacology and Physiology, University of Missouri,
1 Hospital Drive, Rm. MA 415, Columbia, MO 65212, USA
e-mail: sowag@health.missouri.edu

I. Mercier et al. (eds.), *Caveolins in Cancer Pathogenesis, Prevention and Therapy*,
Current Cancer Research, DOI 10.1007/978-1-4614-1001-0_6,
© Springer Science+Business Media, LLC 2012

It has been hypothesized that the balance between pro-angiogenic and anti-angiogenic factors governs the angiogenic switch [2]. According to this hypothesis, the angiogenic switch shifts the balance toward angiogenesis by either inducing pro-angiogenic or by inhibiting anti-angiogenic factors.

The most prominent pro-angiogenic factors are the vascular endothelial growth factor (VEGF) and the fibroblast growth factor (FGF) family. VEGF induces both EC proliferation and migration, which are key steps for angiogenesis [4]. The FGF family of growth factors consists of basic FGF (bFGF, FGF2) and acidic FGF (aFGF, FGF1) [5, 6]. The expression of VEGF receptor (VEGFR) is restricted to ECs on blood and lymphatic vessels, whereas FGF and FGFR are expressed in various cell types. Another factor reported to have pro-angiogenic activity is platelet-derived growth factor B (PDGF-B). PDGF-B induces proliferation and migration of smooth muscle cells and pericytes and can upregulate expression of VEGF and VEGFR2 in cardiac ECs [7, 8]. An additional group of pro-angiogenic factors are the angiopoietins. Although angiopoietins cannot affect EC proliferation per se, they play an important role in the development of newly formed vessels. Angiopoietin-1 promotes recruitment of pericytes and smooth muscle cells and blood vessel maturation. Angiopoietin-2 may antagonize Angiopoietin-1 activity, and its expression is often up-regulated prior to vessel sprouting [9]. The combined action of pro-angiogenic factors initiates and maintains the tumor-associated angiogenesis. In this process, the pro-angiogenic factors VEGF, FGF, PDGF, and angiopoietins play distinct roles. In other words, different stages of angiogenesis, such as initiation and maintenance are regulated by different pro-angiogenic factors. For example, both VEGF and FGF act directly on ECs, by stimulating proliferation and migration. However, it appears that VEGF predominantly affects the initiation of angiogenesis, while FGF regulates the maintenance of tumor angiogenesis [10].

ECs, which are a key player in tumor angiogenesis, respond to numerous different growth factors, cytokines, and chemokines. Certain pro-angiogenic factors can make ECs more responsive to additional pro-angiogenic factors. For example, stimulation of ECs with FGF2 results in the up-regulated expression of VEGFR2, and VEGF-A can up-regulate FGF-R expression. In addition, VEGF-A and FGF2 can synergistically promote angiogenesis through enhancement of endogenous PDGF-B signaling [11]. Also, angiopoietin-2 may render ECs responsive to additional angiogenic factors such as VEGF-A to induce proliferation, migration, and tube formation, or to prevent apoptosis. Conversely, angiopietin-1 has been found to induce maturation and to inhibit leakiness of the endothelium by reducing its responsiveness to angiogenic factors [12, 13].

Caveolins

A more extensive overview of caveolins and their function can be found in many excellent review articles [14–17]. In brief, caveolins are key protein components of detergent resistant and cholesterol lipid rich membranes including lipid rafts and caveolae. There are three members within the caveolin protein family: Caveolin-1 (Cav-1), Cav-2, and Cav-3 [18]. Cav-1 and -2 are co-expressed in most cell types and tissues, while Cav-3 is muscle-specific [18]. The functions of caveolins and caveolae are potentially diverse, as they are capable of regulating multiple signaling transduction pathways in various cell/tissue types [14–17]. Although direct data supporting the role of Cav-2 and -3 in tumor-induced angiogenesis is currently lacking, there is a large body of evidence suggesting positive or negative role for Cav-1 in tumor-induced angiogenesis. The purpose of this chapter is to summarize and where possible, reconcile the existing body of literature involving both basic in vivo and in vitro data as well as correlative clinical evidence pointing at the importance of caveolins, in particular Cav-1 in regulating tumor-induced angiogenesis.

Evidence Supporting a Positive Role of Cav-1 in Tumor Angiogenesis

Many independent studies using mouse models of tumor-induced angiogenesis coupled with Cav-1 knockout (KO) or overexpression approaches in vivo as well as more mechanistic data obtained using in vitro angiogenesis assays and relevant to angiogenesis EC signaling provided compelling evidence for a positive role of Cav-1 in tumor angiogenesis. These basic research data are further supported by independent clinical studies positively associating Cav-1 expression with tumor microvascular density (MVD) and progression.

Positive Role of Cav-1 in Mouse Models of Tumor Growth and Tumor-Induced Angiogenesis

A positive role of Cav-1 in tumor-induced angiogenesis in vivo has been reported using mouse B16 melanoma and RM-9 prostate cancer cells implanted in Cav-1 KO and wild type (WT) C57BL/6 mice or human prostate cancer LNCaP cells implanted into nude mice (see Table 6.1).

Woodman et al. [19] provided the first genetic evidence for a pro-angiogenic function of host cell-expressed Cav-1 in tumor-induced angiogenesis in vivo. In these studies, the melanoma cell line, B16-F10 was subcutaneously (s.c.) injected into C57BL/6 WT and Cav-1 KO mice. The results of these studies revealed that tumor weight, volume, and vessel density determined from hematoxylin and eosin-stained paraffin-embedded sections were all reduced in Cav-1 KO relative to WT mice.

Consistently, a more recent study, using a similar model of tumor-induced angiogenesis involving s.c. implantation of B16-F1 melanoma cells [20], also reported largely reduced tumor growth in Cav-1 KO relative to WT mice. This limited tumor growth in Cav-1 KO mice was associated with diminished angiogenesis determined by counting EC-specific marker CD31-positive structures with lumens [20].

Table 6.1 Pro and anti-angiogenic role of Cav-1 in various models of tumor-induced angiogenesis in vivo

In vivo models of tumor angiogenesis	Pro-angiogenic function of Cav-1	Anti-angiogenic function of Cav-1
Subcutaneous injection of mouse B16-F1 melanoma cells	Reduced tumor weight and angiogenesis in Cav-1 KO mice [20]	
Subcutaneously injection of B16-F10 melanoma tumors in vivo	Reduced tumor weight, volume, and vessel density in Cav-1 KO mice [19]	Faster tumor growth, higher density of CD31-positive vascular structures, increase in blood plasma volume and fibrinogen accumulation in Cav-1 KO mice [33]
Subcutaneous injection of mouse Lewis lung carcinoma cells		Delayed tumor growth, impaired NO-dependent tumor blood flow, and decreased CD31-positive tumor microvessel density upon administration of Cav-1 DNA-lipocomplex in tumor-bearing mice [31]
		Faster tumor growth rate, increased tumor angiogenesis, tumor vascular permeability in Cav-1 KO mice. Administration of cavtratin, a Cav-1 mimetic peptide, corrected the tumor hyperpermeability and attenuated the increased tumor growth [32]
Orthotopic prostate injection of mouse RM-9 cells	Reduced tumor weight and density of CD31-positive microvessels in Cav-1 KO mice	
Subcutaneous injection of human prostate cancer cells (LNCaP) in nude mice	Increased tumor volumes and CD31 positive tumor microvessel density upon doxycycline-induced expression of Cav-1 in LNCaP tumors [21]	

Comprehensive in vivo and in vitro evidence supporting a pro-angiogenic role for Cav-1 has recently been presented in another study [21] using an orthotopic RM-9 mouse prostate cancer model. Specifically, Cav-1 expressing and secreting RM-9 prostate cancer cells were injected directly into the dorsolateral prostate of male WT or Cav-1 KO mice. As in other studies, the mean tumor wet weight and density of CD31 positive microvessels were significantly reduced in Cav-1 KO relative to WT mice. Interestingly, a majority of the CD31 positive microvessels in the Cav-1 KO mouse tumor sections were also positive for Cav-1 staining, indicating uptake of tumor cell-derived Cav-1 by tumor-associated ECs [21]. The role of tumor cell-expressed and secreted Cav-1 was addressed further with a human prostate cell line, LNCaP, in which Cav-1 expression could be induced with doxycycline. Interestingly, both tumor volumes and tumor microvessel density were significantly greater in nude mice implanted s.c. with LNCaP cells, when tumor cell expression of Cav-1 was induced with doxycyclin, suggesting that Cav-1 expression in the prostate cancer cells themselves also plays a pro-angiogenic role [21].

Positive Role of Cav-1 in In Vitro Assays of Angiogenesis

Results of multiple in vitro studies involving EC proliferation, migration, capillary tube formation/differentiation in matrigel, invasion, and angiogenesis-associated signaling, pointing toward a pro-angiogenic role of Cav-1, have been reported within the past few years (see Table 6.2).

For example, ECs isolated from aortas of Cav-1 KO mice displayed defective VEGF-stimulated NO production and tube formation in matrigel relative to WT counterparts [22]. Mechanistically, VEGF-treated Cav-1 KO ECs exhibited impaired phosphorylation of endothelial nitric oxide synthase (eNOS) at Ser1177 and dephosphorylation at Thr495, as well as impaired Erk phosphorylation. Transfection of Cav-1 into Cav-1 KO ECs restored the VEGFR2 targeting to caveolar membranes and the VEGF-induced Erk and eNOS activation [22].

Another study involving aortic ECs from WT and Cav-1 KO mice and recombinant Cav-1 [21] determined that recombinant Cav-1 taken up by ECs through either a lipid raft/caveolae- or clathrin-dependent mechanism could also restore specific angiogenic activities such as tube formation in matrigel, cell migration, and NO production in Cav-1 KO ECs. Specifically, although the formation of tubes in matrigel was reduced in Cav-1 KO ECs relative to WT, treatment with recombinant Cav-1 stimulated tube formation in Cav-1 KO ECs in a dose-dependent manner. Recombinant Cav-1 treatment also stimulated Cav-1 KO EC migration in an in vitro wound healing assay and increased phosphorylation of Akt at Ser473 and Thr308 and subsequent eNOS phosphorylation at Ser1177 but not Thr495, leading to NO production [21].

Multiple studies using antisense or siRNA approaches, often coupled with Cav-1 overexpression, provided independent evidence supporting pro-angiogenic role of Cav-1 in vitro. For instance, knockdown of Cav-1 with antisense oligos resulted in

Table 6.2 Pro- and anti-angiogenic role of Cav-1 based on various angiogenesis assays and relevant EC signaling in vitro

In vitro assays of angiogenesis, EC signaling or Cav-1 expression level	Indicator of pro-angiogenic function of Cav-1	Indicator of anti-angiogenic function of Cav-1
EC proliferation in vitro		Decreased VEGF-stimulated proliferation and S phase transition in HUVEC overexpressing Cav-1 [35]
EC migration in vitro	Cyclodextrin decreased VEGF-stimulated directional migration of bovine aortic ECs [37]	Increased Sphingosine-1-phosphate-stimulated directional migration of bovine aortic ECs treated with Cav-1 siRNA [52]
	HUVEC treated with cyclodextrin, filipin or Cav-1 siRNA have impaired migration [25]	
	VEGF-stimulated directional migration of HUVEC is suppressed by Cav-1 siRNA [26]	
	Enhanced Cav-1 KO aortic EC migration in an in vitro wound healing assay by treatment with recombinant Cav-1 [21]	
Invasion into collagen gel in vitro	Cyclodextrin, filipin, or Cav-1 siRNA inhibit the invasion of HUVEC [25]	
Capillary-like tube formation on matrigel in vitro	Increased capillary-like tube formation of human dermal microvascular ECs upon treatment with adenovirus expressing Cav-1 or with a cell-permeable peptide containing the Cav-1 scaffolding domain. Down-regulation of Cav-1 expression, via an antisense adenoviral approach, reduced the number of capillary-like tubes on matrigel [24]	
	Blocked capillary-like tube formation of HUVEC treated with cyclodextrin, filipin or Cav-1 siRNA [25]	
	Defective capillary tube formation of Cav-1 KO aortic ECs [22]	
	Defective capillary tube formation of Cav-1 KO aortic ECs and dose dependent stimulation upon treatment with recombinant Cav-1 [21]	

Capillary-like tube formation in 3-D fibrin gel in vitro	Suppressed capillary tube formation in HUVEC treated with Cav-1 antisense [23]	
EC signaling	Mislocalized VEGFR2 from caveolar membranes in Cav-1 KO aortic ECs. Transfection of Cav-1 in Cav-1 KO ECs redirected the VEGFR-2 to caveolar membranes [22]	Inhibited VEGFR2 activity by Cav-1 overexpression in 293 cells overexpressing constitutively active VEGFR2 [37]
	Defective VEGF-stimulated Ser1177 eNOS phosphorylation and Thr495 dephosphorylation as well as ERK phosphorylation and NO production in Cav-1 KO aortic ECs. Transfection of Cav-1 in Cav-1 KO ECs restored the VEGF-induced ERK and eNOS activation [22]	More robust and sustained VEGF-stimulated VEGFR2 tyrosine phosphorylation in Cav-1 KO lung ECs. Decreased basal and VEGF-stimulated association between VEGFR2 and the VE-cadherin complex in Cav-1 KO lung ECs [32]
	Increased phosphorylation of Akt at Ser473 and Thr308 and subsequent eNOS phosphorylation of Ser1177 but not Thr495, leading to NO production in Cav-1 KO aortic ECs treated with recombinant Cav-1 [21]	Increased VEGFR3 autophosphorylation in Cav-1 siRNA transfected ECs [38]
		Reduced basal NO release/eNOS activity in cells treated with a cell permeable peptide containing the Cav-1 scaffolding domain or adenoviral overexpression of Cav-1 [41–43]
		Decreased activity of VEGFR2 and down-stream p42/44 MAP kinase in HUVEC overexpressing Cav-1 upon adenoviral delivery [35]
Cav-1 expression level	Increased Cav-1 expression during capillary-like tube formation on matrigel by human dermal microvascular ECs [24]	Reduced Cav-1 expression in ECV 304 cells treated with pro-angiogenic factors such as VEGF, bFGF, or HGF. Treatment with anti-angiogenic factors such as angiostatin, fumagillin, 2-methoxy estradiol, TGF-beta, and thalidomide blocked VEGF-induced down-regulation of Cav-1 [34]
		Reduced Cav-1 expression in brain ECs by pro-angiogenic factors treatment, hypoxia or co-culture with tumor cells and reduced Cav-1 expression in ECs isolated from gliomas with a concurrent increase in tyrosine 14 phosphorylation of Cav-1 [36]

suppression of capillary tube formation by human umbilical vein EC (HUVEC) in fibrin gel-based 3D-angiogenesis assay [23]. Cav-1 has been shown to positively regulate capillary-like tube formation in an in vitro matrigel assay using human dermal microvascular ECs [24]. Specifically, the authors observed an increased level of Cav-1 expression during tube formation in matrigel with the maximum level of Cav-1 expression occurring just prior to the formation of capillary-like tubes. Adenoviral overexpression of Cav-1 enhanced EC differentiation/tubule formation, while down-regulation of Cav-1 expression via an antisense adenoviral approach reduced the number of capillary-like tubes. Consistent with adenoviral overexpression of Cav-1, treatment with a cell permeable peptide containing the Cav-1 scaffolding domain also enhanced capillary-like tube formation [24].

Treatment with the two caveolae-disrupting agents cyclodextrin and filipin or selective targeting of Cav-1 expression with siRNA resulted in blocking MT1-MMP function and inhibition of PMA-stimulated HUVEC migration through polycarbonate filters and invasion into type I collagen gel as well as capillary tube formation in matrigel [25]. Similarly, siRNA-mediated knockdown of Cav-1 inhibited directional cell migration in HUVEC stimulated with VEGF in a Dunn chamber assay, demonstrating that Cav-1 is crucial for VEGF-induced migration [26].

Correlative Evidence Supporting a Positive Role of Cav-1 in Tumor Angiogenesis Based on Clinical Studies

A considerable amount of evidence has accumulated correlating Cav-1 expression with tumor MVD in humans (See Table 6.3).

For instance, double immunohistochemical staining with specific antibodies against Cav-1- and EC-specific marker CD34 of formalin-fixed, paraffin-embedded clear cell renal cell carcinoma tissue sections from 67 patients undergoing radical nephrectomy was performed by Joo et al. [27]. These studies determined a good correlation between MVD and Cav-1 intensity. Further, the Cav-1 proportion and CD34 positive MVD were significantly correlated with the degree of metastasis. The survival of patients with higher Cav-1 intensity in tumor sections was significantly worse than that of patients with lower Cav-1 intensity [27]. These data suggest that Cav-1 plays a pro-angiogenic role in the progression of clear cell renal carcinoma, leading to poor clinical prognosis for patients whose cancer cells express higher levels of Cav-1.

Using double immunofluorescent labeling with antibodies to CD34 and Cav-1, it has been determined that the MVD values were also significantly higher in Cav-1-positive than in Cav-1-negative prostate cancer tumors [28]. Interestingly, Cav-1 positivity in microvessels within tumor specimens was significantly less frequent than in the blood vessels of benign prostatic tissues. In contrast, the percentage of Cav-1-positive tumor associated ECs in Cav-1-positive tumors was significantly higher than in Cav-1-negative tumors. This increased Cav-1 positivity in tumor-associated ECs was predominantly confined to regions with Cav-1-positive tumor cells,

Table 6.3 Clinical correlation of Cav-1 expression with tumor microvascular density (MVD)

Tumor type	Positive (+) or negative (−) correlation of Cav-1 expression with increased MVD	References
Clear cell renal cell carcinoma	+	[27]
Prostate cancer	+	[28]
Meningioma	+	[29]
Hepatic cell carcinoma	+	[30]
Mucoepidermoid carcinoma of the salivary glands	−	[44]

corresponding to the higher percentage of Cav-1-positive microvessels within these regions, as opposed to Cav-1-negative tumors. These data suggest that prostate cancer cell-derived Cav-1 could be involved in mediating angiogenesis during prostate cancer progression in humans [28].

Double immunohistochemical staining with Cav-1 and a tumor EC-specific marker (CD105) antibodies in formalin-fixed, paraffin-embedded human meningioma sections revealed that Cav-1 expression in tumor cells strongly correlated with a significantly higher MVD, suggesting pro-angiogenic function of Cav-1 during meningioma progression in humans [29].

Using dual-label immunofluorescence staining with Cav-1 and CD34 antibodies on formalin-fixed, paraffin-embedded tissue sections of hepatocellular carcinoma, it has been recently determined that Cav-1 expression correlated positively with MVD, suggesting that Cav-1 plays a positive role in regulating hepatic cell carcinoma tumor-induced angiogenesis in humans [30].

Evidence Supporting a Negative Role of Cav-1 in Tumor Angiogenesis

Evidence pointing at a negative role of Cav-1 in tumor angiogenesis based on in vivo and in vitro models of angiogenesis has also accumulated in recent years [31–43]. However, little clinical evidence supporting a negative role of tumor cell expressed Cav-1 in tumor angiogenesis in humans has been obtained to date.

Negative Role of Cav-1 in Mouse Models of Tumor Growth and Tumor-Induced Angiogenesis

Negative role of Cav-1 in tumor-induced angiogenesis in vivo has been reported using Cav-1 KO mice as well as Cav-1 overexpression or delivery of cell-permeable peptide containing Cav-1 scaffolding domain in vivo (Table 6.1). For example, transfection of the liposome Cav-1 plasmid complex through the tail vein of s.c. implanted Lewis lung carcinoma (LLC) cells tumor-bearing WT C57BL mice resulted in a dramatic tumor growth delay [31]. Curiously, using laser Doppler imaging and microprobes, in the early time after introduction of the liposome Cav-1 plasmid complex, when macroscopic effects on the integrity of the tumor vasculature were not yet detectable Cav-1 expression impaired NO-dependent tumor blood flow. At later stages, a decrease in CD31 positive tumor microvessel density in the central core of Cav-1 transfected tumors was also observed [31]. These data suggest an inhibitory effect of overexpressed Cav-1 in regulating tumor-induced angiogenesis, particularly during later stages of tumor growth.

The first genetic evidence for a negative role of Cav-1 in tumor-induced angio-genesis was provided by Lin et al. [32]. Specifically, to address whether the loss of host Cav-1 affects tumor growth, LLC cells were implanted into both WT and Cav-1 KO mice and tumor growth was monitored over time. LLC implanted into Cav-1 KO mice grew faster than in WT mice. This significantly higher tumor growth rate was attributable to increased tumor angiogenesis in Cav-1 KO implanted tumors as determined by immunofluorescent staining of microvessels with anti-VE-cadherin and CD31 antibodies on frozen tumor sections. This increased microvessel density observed in tumor bearing Cav-1 KO mice was also associated with decreased tumor cell death as determined by TUNEL staining. There was no change in tumor cell proliferation as revealed by immunohistochemical staining with Ki-67 antibody. In addition to increased angiogenesis, Cav-1 KO mice displayed increased tumor vascular permeability, measured by Evans blue extravasation and fibrinogen depo-sition compared with tumors implanted into WT mice. Furthermore, administration of a cell permeable peptide containing the scaffolding domain of Cav-1 through the tail vein of Cav-1 KO mice was able to correct the tumor vascular hyperpermeability as well as attenuate the increased tumor growth. Interestingly, despite faster growth rate, increased angiogenesis, and permeability, LLC tumors implanted in the Cav-1 KO mice had significantly lower levels of VEGF measured by ELISA [32]. Overall, this data suggest that Cav-1 is an anti-angiogenic factor in LLC model of tumor-induced angiogenesis.

In their studies, Dewever et al. [33] used s.c. implanted B16-F10 melanoma bearing Cav-1 KO and WT mice to examine the role of host expressed Cav-1 in the regulation of tumor growth, angiogenesis, and vascular permeability. These studies demonstrated an increase in blood plasma volume in Cav-1 KO tumors by dynamic contrast enhanced-magnetic resonance imaging, which was found to be associated with a more rapid tumor growth. Immunostaining analyses of Cav-1 KO tumor sections further revealed a higher density of CD31-positive vascular structures, suggesting increased angiogenesis. They also found that fibrinogen, a readout of avascular per-meability, accumulated in early-stage tumors to a larger extent in Cav-1 KO than in WT mice. These results were confirmed by the observations of a net elevation of the interstitial fluid pressure and a relative deficit in albumin extravasation in Cav-1 KO tumors (vs. healthy tissues) [33]. Mural cell coverage of tumor microvasculature was also examined in these studies. Interestingly, a dramatic deficit in alpha-smooth muscle actin-stained mural cells was observed. An in vitro wound assay and the aortic ring assay revealed that siRNA knockdown of Cav-1 expression could directly impair the migration of smooth muscle cells/pericytes, particularly in response to PDGF [33]. This data suggests that Cav-1 may suppress tumor-induced angiogenesis and promote its termination by increasing mural cell recruitment.

Negative Role of Cav-1 in In Vitro Assays of Angiogenesis

Several pieces of evidence based on in vitro assays pointing toward a negative role of Cav-1 in angiogenesis have also been reported. Many of these studies have examined the role and expression of Cav-1 in EC proliferation in vitro. In their studies, Liu et al. [34] have shown that treatment of ECV 304 cells with known angiogenic growth factors VEGF, bFGF, or HGF resulted in a dramatic reduction in the expression of Cav-1. A variety of angiogenesis inhibitors including angiostatin, fumagillin, 2-methoxy estradiol, TGF-beta, and thalidomide effectively blocked VEGF-induced down-regulation of Cav-1 [34]. This data suggests that Cav-1 may potentially inhibit VEGF-stimulated EC proliferation. A follow up study involving overexpression of Cav-1 in HUVEC confirmed the latter hypothesis [35]. Specifically, adenoviral overexpression of Cav-1 dramatically inhibited the proliferation of HUVEC in response to VEGF as well as the kinase activity of VEGFR2 and the down-stream p42/44 MAP kinase [35].

In their studies, Regina et al. [36] have shown that in brain ECs, Cav-1 is down-regulated by angiogenic factors treatment and by hypoxia or co-culture with tumor cells. They also purified ECs from gliomas as well as from normal brain to investigate possible regulation of Cav-1 expression in tumor brain vasculature. Interestingly, Cav-1 expression was strikingly down-regulated in glioma ECs alone with a concurrent increase in tyrosine-14 phosphorylation of Cav-1. The authors concluded that the down-regulation of Cav-1 expression in tumor ECs may reflect the tumor vasculature state and correlates with angiogenesis kinetics [36].

Using immunoprecipitation of bovine aortic EC lysates, Labrecque et al. [37] have shown that the kinetics of Cav-1 dissociation from VEGFR2 complex correlated with a VEGF-dependent VEGFR2 tyrosine phosphorylation, suggesting that Cav-1 acts as a negative regulator of VEGFR2 activity. In an overexpression system in which VEGFR2 was constitutively active, Cav-1 overexpression inhibited VEGFR2 activity [37].

Lin et al. [32] performed mechanistic studies on lung ECs isolated from Cav-1 KO and WT mice to explain how Cav-1 deficiency in the tumor vasculature could contribute to the observed increased tumor angiogenesis and permeability in vivo. They observed that in Cav-1 KO ECs, VEGF-stimulated VEGFR2 tyrosine phosphorylation was more robust and sustained compared with WT ECs. Because VEGFR2 has been previously reported to associate with proteins from the adherens junction such as VE-cadherin and beta-catenin that negatively regulate the tyrosine phosphorylation of VEGFR2, they examined whether the increased tyrosine phosphorylation of VEGFR2 seen in Cav-1 KO ECs could also be attributed to its lack of association with VE-cadherin. Indeed, a decreased basal and VEGF-stimulated association between VEGFR2 and the VE-cadherin complex were observed in the Cav-1 KO ECs compared with WT ECs. Thus the loss of Cav-1 may enhance VEGFR2 phosphorylation via reduced association with VE-cadherin, which could potentially explain increased eNOS-dependent tumor vessel permeability and angiogenesis observed in Cav-1 KO mice [32].

In addition to VEGFR2, most recent data also suggests that Cav-1 could also be a negative regulator of VEGFR3 activation, i.e., Cav-1 silencing with siRNA increased VEGFR3 autophosphorylation in ECs, suggesting an inhibitory role of Cav-1 on VEGFR3 activities in angiogenesis and lymphangiogenesis [38].

Using coimmunoprecipitation and domain-mapping studies, several laboratories have shown that eNOS, which is one of the downstream signaling mediators for VEGFR2, directly interacts with the scaffolding domain of Cav-1 (residues 82–101) [39, 40]. Evidence supporting a functional significance of this interaction in intact cells has been shown by delivery of a cell permeable peptide containing the scaffolding domain of Cav-1 or by adenoviral overexpression of Cav-1 in living cells or tissues. In all instances, NO release was attenuated, consistent with a negative role of Cav-1 in regulating eNOS activity [41–43].

Correlative Evidence for a Negative Role of Cav-1 in Tumor Angiogenesis Based on Clinical Studies

In contrast to the pro-angiogenic role of Cav-1, little clinical evidence is available with regard to potential negative role of tumor cell expressed Cav-1 in tumor-induced angiogenesis in humans. In one report, Shi et al. [44] performed immunohistochemical study to determine the expression levels of Cav-1 and VEGF and the intratumoral microvessel density (labeled by CD34) in patients with mucoepidermoid carcinoma of the salivary glands. These studies revealed inverse correlation between increased MVD and the expression levels of Cav-1 in tumor microvasculature, suggesting that reduced expression of Cav-1 and increased MVD may indicate a poor prognosis for certain patients [44].

Which Factors Could Be Responsible for the Pro- and Anti-angiogenic Roles of Cav-1?

How could Cav-1 play opposite roles in different or even the same models of tumor angiogenesis? It is important to bear in mind that tumor-induced angiogenesis is a function of the delicate balance between many pro- and anti-angiogenic factors, which varies depending on the specific tumor model, stage of tumor growth and angiogenesis, and the genetic background or age of the animals used. Also, differences in specific in vitro assays of angiogenesis along with the source of ECs or choice of pro-angiogenic stimuli may result in different outcomes. The variability among the above mentioned and possibly other less defined factors could contribute to differences observed by various investigators. Importantly, Cav-1 through its scaffolding domain has been shown to interact with and inhibit the activity of several signaling molecules such as eNOS, PI3K, Src, PKC, or Erk, which could play a role in tumor-induced angiogenesis (see review by [14]). Thus, in the absence or presence of low level of pro-angiogenic stimuli, Cav-1 could play an anti-angiogenic role. The switch from anti-to pro-angiogenic function for Cav-1 could take place upon reaching a critical level of pro-angiogenic stimulation, at which point, proper caveolar localization of a pro-angiogenic receptor and/or post-receptor signaling molecule may be necessary for optimal signaling. The latter is due to the fact that Cav-1 is essential for maintaining intact and functional caveolar membranes, which concentrate many receptors and downstream signaling molecules involved in angiogenesis such as VEGFR2 [22, 37], PDGF receptor, Src, eNOS, PI3K, or PKC (reviewed by [45]). Perhaps the best example of such a complex role for Cav-1 vs. proper caveolar localization is the well characterized suppression of basal eNOS activity by Cav-1 and the promotion of agonist-induced stimulation of eNOS through proper caveolar localization, referred to as "the caveolar paradox" (reviewed in [46]).

Does Cav-2 or -3 Play a Role in Tumor Angiogenesis?

Presumably due to strictly muscle, glial, and peripheral nerve-specific expression of Cav-3 [47], no data suggesting involvement of Cav-3 in tumor angiogenesis have so far been reported. However, unlike Cav-3, Cav-2 is ubiquitously co-expressed with Cav-1 and is particularly abundant in ECs. A potential role for Cav-2 in ECs and tumor angiogenesis is thus certainly plausible. Although no direct evidence supporting a role for Cav-2 in regulating tumor angiogenesis is available, there are a few reports involving studies on Cav-2 KO mice and Cav-2 ECs that suggest a possible role for Cav-2 in regulating physiological angiogenesis in the lung and perhaps also pathological angiogenesis in vivo. For example, studies of Woodman et al. [19] revealed more hematoxylin/eosin positive structures in bFGF loaded matrigel plugs implanted in Cav-2 KO relative to WT mice, suggesting enhanced bFGF-induced angiogenesis in the absence of Cav-2. This data implies that Cav-2 is involved in regulating postnatal pathological angiogenesis in vivo.

Razani et al. [48] have observed a hyperproliferative phenotype in the lung of Cav-2 KO mice involving FLK-1+ VEGFR2 + cells. Because Flk-1 is widely believed to be predominantly expressed in mouse ECs, this observation suggests that Cav-2 may regulate EC proliferation and physiological angiogenesis in the lung. In a most recent study, using pure populations of lung ECs isolated from Cav-2 KO and WT mice, we have determined that Cav-2 directly suppresses EC proliferation [49], suggesting a potential for Cav-2 to affect tumor-induced angiogenesis through regulating EC proliferation. In addition, the fact that Cav-2 can be serine phosphorylated

[50] and that serine 36 phosphorylation of Cav-2 increases in mitotic ECs [51] provides some mechanistic insights as to how Cav-2 could regulate EC proliferation and potentially tumor angiogenesis. However, direct studies comparing tumor growth and tumor-induced angiogenesis in Cav-2 KO vs. WT mice using appropriate in vivo models will be required to determine if Cav-2 actually plays a role in tumor-induced angiogenesis.

Conclusion

Overwhelming evidence has accumulated suggesting that Cav-1 regulates tumor angiogenesis based on in vivo mouse models and in vitro assays of angiogenesis as well as clinical studies. Although the results from mouse models of tumor angiogenesis and relevant in vitro angiogenesis assays are nearly evenly divided between pro- and anti-angiogenic function of Cav-1, the prevailing clinical data favor a positive role for Cav-1 in angiogenesis associated with growth and progression of several cancer types in humans. Many important questions still remain. For example, exactly why and how Cav-1 could play opposite roles in tumor angiogenesis using different or sometimes the same models of tumor angiogenesis? Clearly, more basic research studies will be required to precisely define the role of Cav-1 during different stages of tumor angiogenesis. Also, studies exploring how Cav-1 regulates pro-angiogenic and anti-angiogenic pathways and factors in addition to VEGF, bFGF, or PDGF will be crucial for a better understanding of Cav-1's role in regulating tumor angiogenesis. In addition, exploring the role of Cav-2, the major interacting partner of Cav-1, in tumor-induced angiogenesis using in vivo models such as B16 melanoma and LLC as well as relevant in vitro assays and associated signaling events will also be of key significance.

Acknowledgments Work in the author's laboratory on this topic is supported by the grant from the National Institute of Health (1R01HL081860 to GS).

References

1. Folkman J (1990) What is the evidence that tumors are angiogenesis dependent? J Natl Cancer Inst 82(1):4–6
2. Hanahan D, Folkman J (1996) Patterns and emerging mechanisms of the angiogenic switch during tumorigenesis. Cell 86(3):353–364
3. Staton CA et al (2004) Current methods for assaying angiogenesis in vitro and in vivo. Int J Exp Pathol 85(5):233–248
4. Lohela M et al (2009) VEGFs and receptors involved in angiogenesis versus lymphangiogenesis. Curr Opin Cell Biol 21(2):154–165
5. Folkman J, Shing Y (1992) Angiogenesis. J Biol Chem 267(16):10931–10934
6. Friesel RE, Maciag T (1995) Molecular mechanisms of angiogenesis: fibroblast growth factor signal transduction. FASEB J 9(10):919–925
7. Cao Y, Cao R, Hedlund EM (2008) R Regulation of tumor angiogenesis and metastasis by FGF and PDGF signaling pathways. J Mol Med 86(7):785–789

8. Edelberg JM et al (1998) PDGF mediates cardiac microvascular communication. J Clin Invest 102(4):837–843
9. Tait CR, Jones PF (2004) Angiopoietins in tumours: the angiogenic switch. J Pathol 204(1):1–10
10. Compagni A et al (2000) Fibroblast growth factors are required for efficient tumor angiogenesis. Cancer Res 60(24):7163–7169
11. Kano MR et al (2005) VEGF-A and FGF-2 synergistically promote neoangiogenesis through enhancement of endogenous PDGF-B-PDGFRbeta signaling. J Cell Sci 118(Pt 16):3759–3768
12. Lobov IB, Brooks PC, Lang RA (2002) Angiopoietin-2 displays VEGF-dependent modulation of capillary structure and endothelial cell survival in vivo. Proc Natl Acad Sci USA 99(17):11205–11210
13. Thurston G et al (2000) Angiopoietin-1 protects the adult vasculature against plasma leakage. Nat Med 6(4):460–463
14. Patel HH, Murray F, Insel PA (2008) Caveolae as organizers of pharmacologically relevant signal transduction molecules. Annu Rev Pharmacol Toxicol 48:359–391
15. Thomas CM, Smart EJ (2008) Caveolae structure and function. J Cell Mol Med 12(3):796–809
16. Mercier I et al (2009) Clinical and translational implications of the caveolin gene family: lessons from mouse models and human genetic disorders. Lab Invest 89(6):614–623
17. Parat MO (2009) The biology of caveolae: achievements and perspectives. Int Rev Cell Mol Biol 273:117–162
18. Williams TM, Lisanti MP (2004) The Caveolin genes: from cell biology to medicine. Ann Med 36(8):584–595
19. Woodman SE et al (2003) Caveolin-1 knockout mice show an impaired angiogenic response to exogenous stimuli. Am J Pathol 162(6):2059–2068
20. Chang SH et al (2009) Vascular permeability and pathological angiogenesis in caveolin-1-null mice. Am J Pathol 175(4):1768–1776
21. Tahir SA et al (2008) Tumor cell-secreted caveolin-1 has proangiogenic activities in prostate cancer. Cancer Res 68(3):731–739
22. Sonveaux P et al (2004) Caveolin-1 expression is critical for vascular endothelial growth factor-induced ischemic hindlimb collateralization and nitric oxide-mediated angiogenesis. Circ Res 95(2):154–161
23. Griffoni C et al (2000) Knockdown of caveolin-1 by antisense oligonucleotides impairs angiogenesis in vitro and in vivo. Biochem Biophys Res Commun 276(2):756–761
24. Liu J et al (2002) Caveolin-1 expression enhances endothelial capillary tubule formation. J Biol Chem 277(12):10661–10668
25. Galvez BG et al (2004) Caveolae are a novel pathway for membrane-type 1 matrix metalloproteinase traffic in human endothelial cells. Mol Biol Cell 15(2):678–687
26. Beardsley A et al (2005) Loss of caveolin-1 polarity impedes endothelial cell polarization and directional movement. J Biol Chem 280(5):3541–3547
27. Joo HJ et al (2004) Increased expression of caveolin-1 and microvessel density correlates with metastasis and poor prognosis in clear cell renal cell carcinoma. BJU Int 93(3):291–296
28. Yang G et al (2007) Correlative evidence that prostate cancer cell-derived caveolin-1 mediates angiogenesis. Hum Pathol 38(11):1688–1695
29. Barresi V, Cerasoli S, Tuccari G (2008) Correlative evidence that tumor cell-derived caveolin-1 mediates angiogenesis in meningiomas. Neuropathology 28(5):472–478
30. Zhang ZB et al (2009) Overexpression of caveolin-1 in hepatocellular carcinoma with metastasis and worse prognosis: correlation with vascular endothelial growth factor, microvessel density and unpaired artery. Pathol Oncol Res 15(3):495–502
31. Brouet A et al (2005) Antitumor effects of in vivo caveolin gene delivery are associated with the inhibition of the proangiogenic and vasodilatory effects of nitric oxide. FASEB J 19(6):602–604
32. Lin MI et al (2007) Caveolin-1-deficient mice have increased tumor microvascular permeability, angiogenesis, and growth. Cancer Res 67(6):2849–2856

33. Dewever J et al (2007) Caveolin-1 is critical for the maturation of tumor blood vessels through the regulation of both endothelial tube formation and mural cell recruitment. Am J Pathol 171(5):1619–1628

34. Liu J et al (1999) Angiogenesis activators and inhibitors differentially regulate caveolin-1 expression and caveolae formation in vascular endothelial cells. Angiogenesis inhibitors block vascular endothelial growth factor-induced down-regulation of caveolin-1. J Biol Chem 274(22):15781–15785

35. Fang K et al (2007) Overexpression of caveolin-1 inhibits endothelial cell proliferation by arresting the cell cycle at G0/G1 phase. Cell Cycle 6(2):199–204

36. Regina A et al (2004) Down-regulation of caveolin-1 in glioma vasculature: modulation by radiotherapy. J Neurosci Res 75(2):291–299

37. Labrecque L et al (2003) Regulation of vascular endothelial growth factor receptor-2 activity by caveolin-1 and plasma membrane cholesterol. Mol Biol Cell 14(1):334–347

38. Galvagni F et al (2007) Vascular endothelial growth factor receptor-3 activity is modulated by its association with caveolin-1 on endothelial membrane. Biochemistry 46(13):3998–4005

39. Garcia-Cardena G et al (1997) Dissecting the interaction between nitric oxide synthase (NOS) and caveolin. Functional significance of the nos caveolin binding domain in vivo. J Biol Chem 272(41):25437–25440

40. Ju H et al (1997) Direct interaction of endothelial nitric-oxide synthase and caveolin-1 inhibits synthase activity. J Biol Chem 272(30):18522–18525

41. Bucci M et al (2000) In vivo delivery of the caveolin-1 scaffolding domain inhibits nitric oxide synthesis and reduces inflammation. Nat Med 6(12):1362–1367

42. Feron O et al (1996) Endothelial nitric oxide synthase targeting to caveolae. Specific interactions with caveolin isoforms in cardiac myocytes and endothelial cells. J Biol Chem 271(37):22810–22814

43. Sowa G, Pypaert M, Sessa WC (2001) Distinction between signaling mechanisms in lipid rafts vs. caveolae. Proc Natl Acad Sci USA 98(24):14072–14077

44. Shi L et al (2007) Expression of caveolin-1 in mucoepidermoid carcinoma of the salivary glands: correlation with vascular endothelial growth factor, microvessel density, and clinical outcome. Cancer 109(8):1523–1531

45. de Laurentiis A, Donovan L, Arcaro A (2007) Lipid rafts and caveolae in signaling by growth factor receptors. Open Biochem J 1:12–32

46. Feron O, Kelly RA (2001) The caveolar paradox: suppressing, inducing, and terminating eNOS signaling. Circ Res 88(2):129–131

47. Gazzerro E et al (2010) Caveolinopathies: from the biology of caveolin-3 to human diseases. Eur J Hum Genet 18(2):137–145

48. Razani B et al (2002) Caveolin-2-deficient mice show evidence of severe pulmonary dysfunction without disruption of caveolae. Mol Cell Biol 22(7):2329–2344

49. Xie L et al (2010) Endothelial cells isolated from Caveolin-2 knockout mice display higher proliferation rate and cell cycle progression relative to their wild type counterparts. Am J Physiol Cell Physiol 298(3):C693–C701

50. Sowa G et al (2003) The phosphorylation of caveolin-2 on serines 23 and 36 modulates caveolin-1-dependent caveolae formation. Proc Natl Acad Sci USA 100(11):6511–6516

51. Sowa G et al (2008) Serine 23 and 36 phosphorylation of caveolin-2 is differentially regulated by targeting to lipid raft/caveolae and in mitotic endothelial cells. Biochemistry 47(1):101–111

52. Gonzalez E et al (2004) Small interfering RNA-mediated down-regulation of caveolin-1 differentially modulates signaling pathways in endothelial cells. J Biol Chem 279(39):40659–40669

Chapter 7
Caveolin-1 and Breast Cancer

Gloria Bonuccelli and Michael P. Lisanti

Introduction

Caveolin-1 (Cav-1), the principal component of caveolae, is a 24-kDa integral plasma membrane protein. It has been proposed that Cav-1 functions as a scaffolding protein [1, 2] to organize and concentrate specific lipids (cholesterol and glyco-sphingolipids) [3–6] and signaling molecules (Src-like kinases, H-Ras, endothelial nitric oxide synthase (eNOS), and G-proteins) [7] within caveolae membranes.

In all cases examined, the Cav-1 scaffolding domain (residues 82–101) interacts with a binding motif present within the catalytic domain of specific signaling molecules to form an inactive complex. Following an appropriate stimulus, Cav-1 is released from the binding motif, causing the propagation of downstream signals. It has been reported that the Cav-1 scaffolding domain inhibits Src family tyrosine kinases (c-Src/Fyn), epidermal growth factor receptor (EGF-R), human epidermal growth factor receptor 2 (HER2/neu), protein kinase C (PKC), and extracellular signal-regulated kinase (ERK) with similar potencies [6, 7].

Caveolae are cellular organelles involved in the pathogenesis of several human diseases [8]. The gene encoding human Cav-1 is localized at the D7S522 locus on human chromosome 7 (7q31.1). Interestingly, D7S522 spans a known common fragile site (FRA7G) that is frequently deleted in a variety of human cancers, including squamous cell carcinomas, prostate cancers, renal cell carcinomas, ovarian, and colon carcinomas as well as breast cancers. These evidences have suggested that Cav-1 may act as a tumor suppressor gene at the D7S522 locus [9].

In fact, the first implication of Cav-1 in cancer was through the experimental observation of its phosphorylation on the Tyrosine-14 residue in v-Src-transformed fibroblasts [10]. In addition, oncogene-mediated transformation of murine NIH-3T3

G. Bonuccelli (✉) • M.P. Lisanti (✉)
Department of Stem Cell Biology & Regenerative Medicine, Thomas Jefferson University,
Philadelphia, PA, USA
e-mail: Gloria.bonuccelli@jefferson.edu; mlisanti@KimmelCancerCenter.org

I. Mercier et al. (eds.), *Caveolins in Cancer Pathogenesis, Prevention and Therapy*,
Current Cancer Research, DOI 10.1007/978-1-4614-1001-0_7,
© Springer Science+Business Media, LLC 2012

fibroblasts resulted in the transcriptional down-regulation of Cav-1 and a loss of identifiable caveolae organelles [11]. A reduction in Cav-1 protein levels and caveolae formation appeared to be common events in transformed cell lines, suggesting that Cav-1 might be "inactivated" during tumorigenesis [12, 13]. Interestingly, Cav-1 expression correlates with cellular adhesion and decreased cell motility [14, 15]. In fact, loss of cell adhesion is a hallmark of cell transformation, since normal cells usually undergo apoptosis in response to cell detachment [16]. Together, these data suggest that a loss of Cav-1 disrupts cellular adhesion and consequently promotes metastasis formation when synergistically combined with uncontrolled cell growth. Finally, it has been reported that the loss of stromal Cav-1 in cancer-associated fibroblasts (CAFs) of breast cancer patients is a crucial predictor of tumor recurrence, metastasis, tamoxifen-resistance, and poor clinical outcome [17].

Role of Cav-1 in Mammary Tumorigenesis

The literature has provided mounting evidences that Cav-1 is down-regulated in many tumors, suggesting its role as a tumor suppressor gene and regulator of proliferative signaling pathways. Indeed, the generation of a Cav-1 knockout (KO) mouse model has provided important insights into the role of Cav-1 in breast cancer [18–20]. Although this model does not show spontaneous mammary tumor formation, it exhibits significant mammary epithelial cell hyperplasia with acini formation and fibrosis [21]. In fact, studies on primary cultures of Cav-1 KO mammary epithelial cells have shown characteristics linked to transformation, such as increased proliferation, growth factor independence, and increased cell invasiveness. These phenotypes were associated with the constitutive activation of ERK-1/2, increased expression of Cyclin D1, and estrogen receptor-α (ERα), as well as signal transducer and activator of transcription 5a (Stat5a) hyper-activation. These pathways are involved in mammary epithelial hyperplasia and tumor initiation [22].

ERK and the classical mitogen-activated protein (MAP) kinase are widely expressed intracellular signaling molecules, which regulate cell proliferation. Defects in the MAP/ERK pathway cause uncontrolled cell growth. In fact, ERK-1/2 can alter the levels and activities of several protein kinases and transcription factors involved in cell cycle, including Elk1, c-Myc, and c-Fos, among others. Interestingly, ERK-1/2 is compartmentalized within caveolae [23, 24] and has been shown to be inhibited by Cav-1 [15, 25]. In particular, a reciprocal negative regulation exists between ERK-1/2 kinase activation and Cav-1 protein expression. For example, up-regulation of Cav-1 protein expression down-modulates ERK-1/2 kinase activity [25], which in turn down-regulates Cav-1 mRNA levels and protein expression [26, 27]. Finally, ERK-1/2 hyper-activation is maintained in vivo as shown in Cav-1 KO mouse tissues [28–30]. Taken together, these findings support a possible role of Cav-1 as a negative regulator of the ERK1/2 signaling pathway.

Cyclin-D1, a protein encoded by the *CCND1* gene in humans, is responsible for the G1 to S phase transition of the cell cycle [31, 32]. The cyclin D1 gene is amplified or over-expressed in almost 50% of human breast cancers [33–36]. This protein has been shown to regulate the activity of the retinoblastoma (Rb) protein. The Rb protein prevents excessive cell growth by inhibiting the cell cycle progression until cells are ready to divide. The cyclin D1 protein forms an active complex that promotes cell cycle progression by phosphorylating and inactivating the Rb protein [37–39]. Cyclin D1 expression is driven by mitogenic and oncogenic signaling pathways and antisense against this cell cycle protein inhibits transformation induced by Ha-ras, Src, and HER2/neu [40–42]. Since caveolae are plasma membrane invaginations with an important role in signal transduction, studies were performed to assess whether Cav-1 could directly regulate cyclin D1 expression. Importantly, in vitro evidences have shown that the cyclin D1 gene is transcriptionally repressed by overexpression of the Cav-1 protein. Full repression of cyclin D1 gene requires the T cell factor/lymphoid enhancer factor-1-binding site (TCF) on its promoter and the Cav-1 N-terminus portion [43]. Thus, inhibition of the cyclin D1 gene by Cav-1 may prevent cellular transformation.

The first demonstration that a loss of Cav-1 promoted mammary tumorigenesis in vivo was provided by a study employing the mouse mammary tumor virus LTR-driven polyoma middle T antigen (MMTV-PyMT) transgenic model interbred with Cav-1 KO mice. Interestingly, mammary tumor samples derived from PyMT/Cav-1 KO mice showed ERK-1/2 hyperactivation, cyclin D1 up-regulation, and increased levels of phospho-Rb [44]. Further studies using Cav-1 KO and MMTV-cyclin D1 transgenic (Tg) mice have provided evidences that Cav-1 functions as an antagonist of cyclin D1 in mammary epithelial cells [45]. In conclusion, these data suggest antiproliferative and transformation-suppressive roles of Cav-1 in mammary epithelial cells.

ERα and ERβ are nuclear proteins that are targets of estrogen actions. Estrogens are important for normal development and maintenance of female characteristics and sexual reproduction. Importantly, while ERα is expressed at low levels in normal mammary epithelial cells, its up-regulation is found in premalignant hyperplasia and during the development of breast carcinomas. Up to one third of human ERα-positive breast cancers harbor Cav-1 mutations [48]. The Cav-1 P132L mutation is found in more than half of estrogen positive breast cancer cases carrying Cav-1 mutations [46, 47]. The Cav-1 (P132L) mutation is caused by a proline to leucine change at position 132 occurring in the putative transmembrane domain of Cav-1 [48]. This mutation leads to ERα overexpression and increased sensitivity toward estrogen, which is an important risk factor for breast tumor development [46, 47]. Recently, studies performed on Cav-1 KO mice, subjected to ovariectomy and estrogen supplementation, supported the evidence that a functional loss of Cav-1 may be sufficient to confer estrogen-hypersensitivity in the mammary gland [49]. In addition, in vitro experiments have shown that overexpression of the Cav-1 (P132L) mutant was sufficient to transform NIH 3T3 cells. Interestingly, the Cav-1 (P132L) mutant was retained in a perinuclear ER/Golgi-like compartment along with endogenous wild type Cav-1 in normal human mammary epithelial cells. Thus, this mutation behaved in a dominant-negative manner since it prevented the proper targeting of wild type Cav-1 to the plasma membrane [21]. To study the behavior of the Cav-1 (P132L) mutation in vivo, the Met-1 cell system was used. The Met-1 cells were obtained from a MMTV-PyMT mammary tumor [50, 51] and have previously been employed to assess the role of Cav-1 (WT) as a tumor suppressor [30]. Recent studies suggest that the Cav-1 (P132L) mutation act as a loss-of-function mutation during primary tumor formation. Interestingly, the Cav-1 (P132L) mutation can also act as a gain-of-function mutation in the context of cell migration, invasion, and experimental metastasis, as shown by DNA microarray studies [52]. Importantly, this new metastasis-associated gene signature could explain why breast cancer patients with a Cav-1 (P132L) mutation are more susceptible to disease recurrence and metastasis formation [52].

In the human breast, prolactin is a major growth and differentiating hormone that binds the transmembrane prolactin receptor (Prl-R). Recently, the formation of this complex has also been recognized as an important mechanism involved in the induction of cell proliferation and progression of mammary tumors. The binding of prolactin to Prl-R causes the recruitment and phosphorylation of Janus kinase 2 (commonly named Jak2), a protein tyrosine kinase implicated in the phosphorylation of Prl-R. Phosphorylated Prl-R activates signaling cascades including the Jak-2/STAT5a, mitogen activated protein kinase (MAPK), and the phosphatidylinositol 3-kinase (PI3K) pathways [53, 54]. Impairment at different levels of the prolactin signaling cascade causes alterations in mammary gland development and lactation.

The first evidence that Cav-1 may function as a negative regulator of the Prl-R/Jak-2/STAT5a signaling cascade in the mammary gland came from studies carried in cultured mammary epithelial cells where Cav-1 overexpression repressed prolactin-induced β-casein transcription [55]. In addition, during late pregnancy and lactation, Cav-1 expression is transcriptionally down-regulated in the mammary gland, but is restored after weaning. Accordingly, female Cav-1 KO mice showed an accelerated mammary development of the lobuloalveolar compartment during pregnancy, with precocious lactation [56]. Lindeman et al [57]. have identified SOCS-1 (suppressor of cytokine signaling-1) as a protein that inhibits Janus kinase/STAT pathway. The Cav-1 scaffolding domain is similar to the SOCS pseudosubstrate domain, which is crucial to inhibit Janus kinases (Jaks). Accordingly, in vitro experiments have demonstrated that Jak2 co-fractionates and co-immunoprecipitates with Cav-1 [56]. Finally, Cav-1 KO mice show a similar premature lactation phenotype as SOCS-1 KO mice. Taken together, these data suggest a role for Cav-1 as a negative regulator of the prolactin signaling axis.

It is well-known that the tumor microenvironment plays an important role in human breast cancer onset and progression. In this regard, the Cav-1 KO mouse was recently showed to be a very useful model to understand the role of Cav-1 in the tumor stroma. It has been shown that human breast CAFs display Cav-1 down-regulation and inactivation of Rb when compared with normal fibroblasts [58]. Importantly, Cav-1 KO mammary stromal fibroblasts (MSFs) share striking similarities with human CAFs in their transcriptional gene profiling and Rb functional inactivation [59]. Thus, Cav-1 KO MSFs may help to understand the signaling pathways activated in the tumor microenvironment.

Role of Cav-1 in Metastasis Formation

During metastasis formation, cellular motility is essential and cancer cells migrate away from the primary tumor site and invade distal tissues. Alterations in cytoskeletal components are responsible for increased motility [60]. Importantly, pro-metastatic growth factors such as the EGF, cause disassembling of actin microfilaments, focal adhesion complexes formation, and form actin-containing lamellipodia and filopodia for migration [61, 62].

To assess whether Cav-1 expression influences the metastatic phenotype of breast cancer cells, studies have been performed both in vitro and in vivo. These have shown that Cav-1 plays a role as a suppressor of breast cancer metastasis [44, 63]. The MMTV-PyMT adenocarcinoma mouse model has been very useful for studying mammary tumor development and metastases formation [64]. By 16 weeks of age, 100% of these transgenic mice develop metastases to the lung, and for this reason, this model represents an exceptional system to study the effect of Cav-1 on metastasis formation. Williams et al. provided the first demonstration that a loss of Cav-1 expression in PyMT/Cav-1 KO mice resulted in increased incidence, frequency, and size of lung metastases derived from mammary adenocarcinomas [44]. Moreover, a role for Cav-1 in the expression and activity of matrix metalloproteinases (MMPs) was also investigated. MMP-2 (gelatinase A) and MMP-9 (gelatinase B) are two well-characterized metalloproteinases secreted by tumor cells, which exhibit collagenolytic and gelatinolytic activities. MMPs activity enhances tumor invasiveness and metastasis formation [65]. Indeed, MMP-2- and MMP-9-deficient mice are much less susceptible to experimental metastasis development [66, 67]. There are currently eight distinct types of MMPs, five of which are secreted and three that are membrane-anchored [68]. Since some MMPs are secreted as inactive zymogens (pro-MMPs), they have to be activated to function. Indeed, there is a membrane-type group, known collectively as MT-MMPs, that not only functions as extracellular matrix degrading enzymes but also serves to activate other MMPs, such as MT1-MMP that activates pro-MMP-2 [69]. Metastatic mammary tumor cells that expressed recombinant Cav-1 showed significant reductions in matrigel invasion and dramatically reduced MMP-9/MMP-2 activities [43]. Several groups have shown that MT1-MMP co-localizes with caveolae and Cav-1 [70–72]. Furthermore, it has been demonstrated that caveolae and Cav-1 are required for proper MT1-MMP localization and activity in migrating endothelial cells [72]. Taken together, these results suggest a potential caveolin-based therapeutic approach for the treatment of metastatic human breast cancer.

Role of Cav-1 in Apoptosis

Apoptosis is a highly programmed type of cell death. The first evidence of a possible role of Cav-1 in the apoptosis process was examined in vitro, in v-Abl and H-Ras (G12V)-transformed NIH 3T3 cells. In this context, Cav-1 re-expression abrogated the anchorage-independent growth of these cells in soft agar, an effect that appeared to be due in part to its ability to initiate apoptosis [73]. In addition, it has been reported that in mouse embryonic fibroblasts and in T24 bladder carcinoma epithelial cells, overexpression of Cav-1 induces apoptotic cell death through inhibition of PI3-kinase and/or activation of caspase-3 [74, 75]. Moreover, recent results from a DNA microarray analysis performed on Met-1 cells [50, 51] overexpressing Cav-1 have revealed the up-regulation of pro-apoptotic genes [52]. Taken together, these results provide evidences that Cav-1 has a pro-apoptotic role. However, it has been shown that up-regulation of Cav-1 in human prostate cancer cells causes resistance to apoptosis, and its antisense down-regulation induces apoptosis [47, 76, 77]. In conclusion, it seems that Cav-1 plays a controversial dual role in the apoptosis process. The apparent incongruity may depend on the cell type or cellular context.

Cav-1 and Tumor Metabolism

Recent studies have proposed a new theory about how cancer cells grow and survive in vivo. This model is based on the original Warburg effect, according to which the tumor metabolism switches from oxidative phosphorylation to aerobic glycolysis to fuel its own growth. The revolutionary difference is that the Warburg effect happens in fibroblasts, not in cancer epithelial cells. For this reason, the new theory that reverts 85 years of dogma is called "the reverse Warburg effect" [78]. CAFs function as supporting cells for cancer progression and provide recycled nutrients to tumor cells. Particularly, cancer cells induce oxidative stress in adjacent CAFs, which mimics the effects of hypoxia causing an over-production of reactive oxygen species (ROS), local DNA damage, and mutations in cancer cells leading to more aggressive tumors [79, 80].

The final effect of oxidative stress is the induction of autophagy and/or mitophagy (the autophagic destruction of mitochondria) in the tumor microenvironment, leading to the stromal production of recycled nutrients, including energy-rich metabolytes like ketones and L-lactate [80–82]. Indeed, CAFs lose their mitochondria via a phenomenon of autophagic destruction and undergo aerobic glycolysis. Aerobic glycolysis of these stromal cells then produces pyruvate, lactate, and ketone bodies (3-hydroxybutyrate) [82] which increases the number of mitochondria in cancer cells, and fuels their TCA cycle and ATP production, accelerating tumor growth and metastasis formation. Finally, it has been shown that oxidative stress also leads to the activation of HIF1-alpha (aerobic glycolysis) and NFkB-(inflammation) in CAFs, causing the onset of autophagy and mitophagy. Taken together, these findings have suggested a new model based on the reverse Warburg effect and on the tumor-stroma co-evolution, named "the autophagic tumor stroma model of cancer cell metabolism".

Clinically, loss of Cav-1 is a predictor of poor prognosis in breast cancer patients, and is linked to early tumor recurrence, lymph node metastasis, and tamoxifen resistance. Importantly, the prognostic value of stromal Cav-1 seems to be independent of other epithelial markers such as ER, PR, HER2 as well as the cancer subtype (basal or

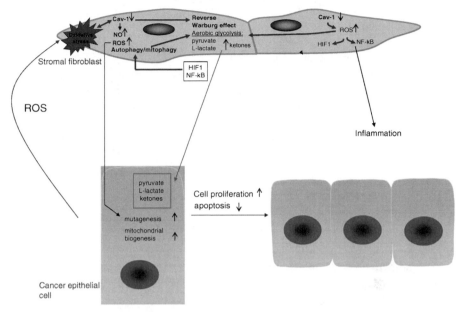

Fig. 7.1 "The autophagic tumor stroma model of cancer cell metabolism." Cancer epithelial cells induce oxidative stress in cancer-associated fibroblasts (CAFs) with over-production of reactive oxygen species (ROS). Importantly, cancer cells induce a loss of Cav-1 and mitochondria in the adjacent fibroblasts. The resulting oxidative stress in stromal fibroblasts leads to tumor-stroma co-evolution, providing cancer cells with abundant recycled nutrients via autophagy/mitophagy, and supplying their oxidative mitochondrial metabolism, the TCA cycle and ATP production. The final effect of the tumor-stroma co-evolution is a random mutagenesis of cancer cells and their protection against apoptosis. Note that the Warburg effect does not occur in the cancer cells but in the stromal fibroblasts, forced to undergo aerobic glycolysis producing pyruvate, lactate and ketone bodies

ductal) [17, 83]. It has been demonstrated that a loss of Cav-1 leads to oxidative stress and mimics hypoxia causing aerobic glycolysis and inflammation in the tumor microenvironment [79, 84]. Importantly, by using Cav-1 deficient stromal cells as a new genetic model of CAFs, the major signaling pathways activated by a loss of Cav-1 have been identified. Indeed, a loss of Cav-1 directly leads to the increase of NO (nitric oxide) production [79, 84], consistent with its role as an endogenous inhibitor of NOS (nitric oxide synthase). In turn, increased NO production generates ROS and oxidative stress through mitochondrial dysfunction with increased tyrosine nitration resulting in the inactivation of mitochondrial complex I [84]. In addition, using an informatics approach such as a transcriptional profiling performed on wild-type and Cav-1 KO mice bone marrow-derived stromal cells, it has been shown that a loss of Cav-1 activated transcription factors such as HIF and NFkB, and caused aerobic glycolysis, inflammation, and angiogenesis in the tumor micro-environment [84, 85].

All of these experimental findings, summarized in Fig. 7.1, have important implications for human breast cancer. This new cancer stromal autophagy theory offers an explanation for the lethal phenotype associated with an absence of stromal Cav-1. In the absence of Cav-1, CAFs from patients with breast cancer are able to feed their cancer epithelial cells with recycled nutrients. In fact, parallel studies in clinical specimens of patients with breast cancer have shown that tumors lacking stromal Cav-1 show stromal overexpression of markers for aerobic glycolysis (PKM2/LDH-B) and mitophagy (BNIP3L) similar to Cav-1KO myofibroblasts and tumors from xenograft model employing MDA-MB-231 human breast cell line [79, 86]. Besides, human samples of breast cancer show increased nitro-tyrosine staining associated with increased VEGF-C expression, lymph node metastasis, and poor clinical outcome [87]. Overall, a loss of stromal Cav-1 is a very good biomarker for identifying high-risk patients.

Conclusions

As we have discussed in this chapter, most research on Cav-1 has been focused on understanding its role in breast cancer. In the tumor epithelium, a mutation of the *Cav-1* gene (P132L) has been identified and shown to directly modulate several signaling pathways involved in cell migration, invasion, and metastasis of breast cancer cells. Importantly, these results may have implications for the diagnostic and therapeutic stratification of human breast cancer. Indeed, genotyping of the primary tumor for Cav-1 mutations could be helpful to identify patients that are more likely to undergo recurrence and/or metastasis [52].

Recent interesting reports have demonstrated that Cav-1 can also regulate tumor associated fibroblasts. In fact, stromal Cav-1 expression has been identified as a new prognostic biomarker for human breast cancer prognosis and therapy [88]. These findings may have important implications for the monitoring and stratification of breast cancer patients. Remarkably, a loss of stromal Cav-1 could also be used to predict ductal carcinoma in situ (DCIS) progression to invasive breast cancer nearly 15–20 years in advance [89]. In addition, more evidences suggest that a role for Cav-1 in the tumor stroma is not restricted to breast cancer patients as similar results have been obtained in prostate cancer patients [90]. Thus, a loss of stromal Cav-1 may be an important prognostic biomarker for other types of cancers besides breast and prostate.

The new proposed theory "tumor-stroma co-evolution," has brought new suggestions for the treatment of breast cancer as well as the re-examination of currently used therapies. One concern is about the common use of lactate before, during, and after surgery in cancer patients. Indeed, the lactate is an energy-rich fuel that increases cancer cell growth and survival. In light of these new studies, this practice should therefore be re-evaluated [81]. Moreover, the new theory suggests that cancer cells do not need blood vessels to feed them [91]. This result explains why some angiogenesis inhibitors have not worked and actually may be dangerous given that effective anti-angiogenic therapies induce hypoxia in the tumor stroma [92–94].

These new studies have suggested the use of novel therapies for breast cancer treatments, which might include the use of antioxidants and autophagy/lysosomal inhibitors to prevent oxidative stress in the tumor fibroblasts, thus cutting off the fuel supply to cancer cells. Importantly, antioxidants like *N*-acetyl-cystein, metformin, and quercetin, as well as lysosomal inhibitors like chloroquine are available as over-the-counter dietary supplements or FDA-approved drugs.

In conclusion, the new roles of Cav-1 in breast cancer both on the cancer epithelium and the tumor stroma will have to be incorporated in patients' diagnosis, stratification, and treatment, which will bring us much closer to perfecting solutions for the treatment of cancer.

References

1. Lisanti MP, Scherer P, Tang Z-L, Sargiacomo M (1994) Caveolae, caveolin and caveolin-rich membrane domains: a signalling hypothesis. Trends Cell Biol 4:231–235
2. Okamoto T, Schlegel A, Scherer PE, Lisanti MP (1998) Caveolins, a family of scaffolding proteins for organizing "pre-assembled signaling complexes" at the plasma membrane. J Biol Chem 273:5419–5422
3. Anderson RGW (1998) The caveolae membrane system. Annu Rev Biochem 67:199–225
4. Brown DA, London E (1998) Functions of lipid rafts in biological membranes. Annu Rev Cell Dev Biol 14:111–136
5. Galbiati F, Razani B, Lisanti MP (2001) Emerging themes in lipid rafts and caveolae. Cell 106:403–411
6. Williams TM, Lisanti MP (2004) The Caveolin genes: from cell biology to medicine. Ann Med 36:584–595
7. Razani B, Woodman SE, Lisanti MP (2002) Caveolae: from cell biology to animal physiology. Pharmacol Rev 54:431–467
8. Mercier I, Jasmin JF, Pavlides S, Minetti C, Flomenberg N, Pestell RG, Frank PG, Sotgia F, Lisanti MP (2009) Clinical and translational implications of the caveolin gene family: lessons from mouse models and human genetic disorders. Lab Invest 89:614–623
9. Engelman JA, Zhang XL, Lisanti MP (1998) Genes encoding human caveolin-1 and -2 are co-localized to the D7S522 locus (7q31.1), a known fragile site (FRA7G) that is frequently deleted in human cancers. FEBS Lett 436:403–410
10. Glenney JR (1989) Tyrosine phosphorylation of a 22 kD protein is correlated with transformation with Rous sarcoma virus. J Biol Chem 264:20163–20166
11. Koleske AJ, Baltimore D, Lisanti MP (1995) Reduction of caveolin and caveolae in oncogenically transformed cells. Proc Natl Acad Sci USA 92:1381–1385
12. Razani B, Altschuler Y, Zhu L, Pestell RG, Mostov KE, Lisanti MP (2000) Caveolin-1 expression is down-regulated in cells transformed by the human papilloma virus in a p53-dependent manner. Replacement of caveolin-1 expression suppresses HPV-mediated cell transformation. Biochemistry 39:13916–13924
13. Engelman JA, Lee RJ, Karnezis A, Bearss DJ, Webster M, Siegel P, Muller WJ, Windle JJ, Pestell RG, Lisanti MP (1998) Reciprocal regulation of Neu tyrosine kinase activity and caveolin-1 protein expression in vitro and in vivo. Implications for mammary tumorigenesis. J Biol Chem 273:20448–20455
14. Volonte D, Galbiati F, Pestell RG, Lisanti MP (2001) Cellular stress induces the tyrosine phosphorylation of caveolin-1 (Tyr(14)) via activation of p38 mitogen-activated protein kinase and c-Src kinase. Evidence for caveolae, the actin cytoskeleton, and focal adhesions as mechanical sensors of osmotic stress. J Biol Chem 276:8094–8103
15. Zhang W, Razani B, Altschuler Y, Bouzahzah B, Mostov KE, Pestell RG, Lisanti MP (2000) Caveolin-1 inhibits epidermal growth factor-stimulated lamellipod extension and cell migration

in metastatic mammary adenocarcinoma cells (MTLn3). Transformation suppressor effects of adenovirus-mediated gene delivery of caveolin-1. J Biol Chem 275:20717–20725
16. Stupack DG, Cheresh DA (2002) Get a ligand, get a life: integrins, signaling and cell survival. J Cell Sci 115:3729–3738
17. Witkiewicz AK, Dasgupta A, Sammons S, Er O, Potoczek MB, Guiles F, Sotgia F, Brody JR, Mitchell EP, Lisanti MP (2010) Loss of stromal caveolin-1 expression predicts poor clinical outcome in triple negative and basal-like breast cancers. Cancer Biol Ther 10:135–143
18. Razani B, Engelman JA, Wang XB, Schubert W, Zhang XL, Marks CB, Macaluso F, Russell RG, Li M, Pestell RG, Di Vizio D, Hou HJ, Kneitz B, Lagaud G, Christ GJ, Edelmann W, Lisanti MP (2001) Caveolin-1 null mice are viable but show evidence of hyperproliferative and vascular abnormalities. J Biol Chem 276:38121–38138
19. Schubert W, Frank PG, Woodman SE, Hyogo H, Cohen DE, Chow CW, Lisanti MP (2002) Microvascular hyperpermeability in caveolin-1 (-/-) knock-out mice. Treatment with a specific nitric-oxide synthase inhibitor, L-NAME, restores normal microvascular permeability in Cav-1 null mice. J Biol Chem 277:40091–40098
20. Drab M, Verkade P, Elger M, Kasper M, Lohn M, Lauterbach B, Menne J, Lindschau C, Mende F, Luft FC, Schedl A, Haller H, Kurzchalia TV (2001) Loss of caveolae, vascular dysfunction, and pulmonary defects in caveolin-1 gene-disrupted mice. Science 293:2449–2452
21. Lee H, Park DS, Razani B, Russell RG, Pestell RG, Lisanti MP (2002) Caveolin-1 mutations (P132L and null) and the pathogenesis of breast cancer: caveolin-1 (P132L) behaves in a dominant-negative manner and caveolin-1 (-/-) null mice show mammary epithelial cell hyperplasia. Am J Pathol 161:1357–1369
22. Sotgia F, Rui H, Bonuccelli G, Mercier I, Pestell RG, Lisanti MP (2006) Caveolin-1, mammary stem cells, and estrogen-dependent breast cancers. Cancer Res 66:10647–10651
23. Liu P, Ying Y, Anderson RG (1997) Platelet-derived growth factor activates mitogen-activated protein kinase in isolated caveolae. Proc Natl Acad Sci USA 94:13666–13670
24. Smart EJ, Ying YS, Mineo C, Anderson RG (1995) A detergent-free method for purifying caveolae membrane from tissue culture cells. Proc Natl Acad Sci USA 92:10104–10108
25. Engelman JA, Chu C, Lin A, Jo H, Ikezu T, Okamoto T, Kohtz DS, Lisanti MP (1998) Caveolin-mediated regulation of signaling along the p42/44 MAP kinase cascade in vivo. A role for the caveolin-scaffolding domain. FEBS Lett 428:205–211
26. Galbiati F, Volonte D, Engelman JA, Watanabe G, Burk R, Pestell RG, Lisanti MP (1998) Targeted down-regulation of caveolin-1 is sufficient to drive cell transformation and hyperactivate the p42/44 MAP kinase cascade. EMBO J 17:6633–6648
27. Engelman JA, Zhang XL, Razani B, Pestell RG, Lisanti MP (1999) p42/44 MAP kinase-dependent and -independent signaling pathways regulate caveolin-1 gene expression. Activation of Ras-MAP kinase and protein kinase a signaling cascades transcriptionally down-regulates caveolin-1 promoter activity. J Biol Chem 274:32333–32341
28. Capozza F, Williams TM, Schubert W, McClain S, Bouzahzah B, Sotgia F, Lisanti MP (2003) Absence of caveolin-1 sensitizes mouse skin to carcinogen-induced epidermal hyperplasia and tumor formation. Am J Pathol 162:2029–2039
29. Cohen AW, Razani B, Wang XB, Combs TP, Williams TM, Scherer PE, Lisanti MP (2003) Caveolin-1-deficient mice show insulin resistance and defective insulin receptor protein expression in adipose tissue. Am J Physiol Cell Physiol 285:C222–C235
30. Williams TM, Lee H, Cheung MW, Cohen AW, Razani B, Iyengar P, Scherer PE, Pestell RG, Lisanti MP (2004) Combined loss of INK4a and caveolin-1 synergistically enhances cell proliferation and oncogene-induced tumorigenesis: role of INK4a/CAV-1 in mammary epithelial cell hyperplasia. J Biol Chem 279:24745–24756
31. Motokura T, Bloom T, Kim HG, Juppner H, Ruderman JV, Kronenberg HM, Arnold A (1991) A novel cyclin encoded by a bcl1-linked candidate oncogene. Nature 350:512–515
32. Lew DJ, Dulic V, Reed SI (1991) Isolation of three novel human cyclins by rescue of G1 cyclin (Cln) function in yeast. Cell 66:1197–1206
33. Lammie GA, Fantl V, Smith R, Schuuring E, Brookes S, Michalides R, Dickson C, Arnold A, Peters G (1991) D11S287, a putative oncogene on chromosome 11q13, is amplified and

expressed in squamous cell and mammary carcinomas and linked to BCL-1. Oncogene 6:439–444

34. Bartkova J, Lukas J, Muller H, Lutzhoft D, Strauss M, Bartek J (1994) Cyclin D1 protein expression and function in human breast cancer. Int J Cancer 57:353–361
35. Gillett C, Fantl V, Smith R, Fisher C, Bartek J, Dickson C, Barnes D, Peters G (1994) Amplification and overexpression of cyclin D1 in breast cancer detected by immunohistochemical staining. Cancer Res 54:1812–1817
36. Sherr CJ (1996) Cancer cell cycles. Science 274:1672–1677
37. Kato J, Matsushime H, Hiebert SW, Ewen ME, Sherr CJ (1993) Direct binding of cyclin D to the retinoblastoma gene product (pRb) and pRb phosphorylation by the cyclin D-dependent kinase CDK4. Genes Dev 7:331–342
38. Lundberg AS, Weinberg RA (1998) Functional inactivation of the retinoblastoma protein requires sequential modification by at least two distinct cyclin-cdk complexes. Mol Cell Biol 18:753–761
39. Sicinski P, Donaher JL, Parker SB, Li T, Fazeli A, Gardner H, Haslam SZ, Bronson RT, Elledge SJ, Weinberg RA (1995) Cyclin D1 provides a link between development and oncogenesis in the retina and breast. Cell 82:621–630
40. Pestell RG, Albanese C, Reutens AT, Segall JE, Lee RJ, Arnold A (1999) The cyclins and cyclin-dependent kinase inhibitors in hormonal regulation of proliferation and differentiation. Endocr Rev 20:501–534
41. Liu JJ, Chao JR, Jiang MC, Ng SY, Yen JJ, Yang-Yen HF (1995) Ras transformation results in an elevated level of cyclin D1 and acceleration of G1 progression in NIH 3T3 cells. Mol Cell Biol 15:3654–3663
42. Lee RJ, Albanese C, Fu M, D'Amico M, Lin B, Watanabe G, Haines GK 3rd, Siegel PM, Hung MC, Yarden Y, Horowitz JM, Muller WJ, Pestell RG (2000) Cyclin D1 is required for transformation by activated Neu and is induced through an E2F-dependent signaling pathway. Mol Cell Biol 20:672–683
43. Hulit J, Bash T, Fu M, Galbiati F, Albanese C, Sage DR, Schlegel A, Zhurinsky J, Shtutman M, Ben-Ze'ev A, Lisanti MP, Pestell RG (2000) The cyclin D1 gene is transcriptionally repressed by caveolin-1. J Biol Chem 275:21203–21209
44. Williams TM, Medina F, Badano I, Hazan RB, Hutchinson J, Muller WJ, Chopra NG, Scherer PE, Pestell RG, Lisanti MP (2004) Caveolin-1 gene disruption promotes mammary tumorigenesis and dramatically enhances lung metastasis in vivo. Role of Cav-1 in cell invasiveness and matrix metalloproteinase (MMP-2/9) secretion. J Biol Chem 279:51630–51646
45. Williams TM, Sotgia F, Lee H, Hassan G, Di Vizio D, Bonuccelli G, Capozza F, Mercier I, Rui H, Pestell RG, Lisanti MP (2006) Stromal and epithelial caveolin-1 both confer a protective effect against mammary hyperplasia and tumorigenesis: caveolin-1 antagonizes cyclin D1 function in mammary epithelial cells. Am J Pathol 169:1784–1801
46. Hayashi K, Matsuda S, Machida K, Yamamoto T, Fukuda Y, Nimura Y, Hayakawa T, Hamaguchi M (2001) Invasion activating caveolin-1 mutation in human scirrhous breast cancers. Cancer Res 61:2361–2364
47. Li L, Ren CH, Tahir SA, Ren C, Thompson TC (2003) Caveolin-1 maintains activated Akt in prostate cancer cells through scaffolding domain binding site interactions with and inhibition of serine/threonine protein phosphatases PP1 and PP2A. Mol Cell Biol 23:9389–9404
48. Li T, Sotgia F, Vuolo MA, Li M, Yang WC, Pestell RG, Sparano JA, Lisanti MP (2006) Caveolin-1 mutations in human breast cancer: functional association with estrogen receptor alpha-positive status. Am J Pathol 168:1998–2013
49. Mercier I, Casimiro MC, Zhou J, Wang C, Plymire C, Bryant KG, Daumer KM, Sotgia F, Bonuccelli G, Witkiewicz AK, Lin J, Tran TH, Milliman J, Frank PG, Jasmin JF, Rui H, Pestell RG, Lisanti MP (2009) Genetic ablation of caveolin-1 drives estrogen-hypersensitivity and the development of DCIS-like mammary lesions. Am J Pathol 174:1172–1190
50. Borowsky AD, Namba R, Young LJ, Hunter KW, Hodgson JG, Tepper CG, McGoldrick ET, Muller WJ, Cardiff RD, Gregg JP (2005) Syngeneic mouse mammary carcinoma cell lines: two closely related cell lines with divergent metastatic behavior. Clin Exp Metastasis 22:47–59

51. Namba R, Young LJ, Abbey CK, Kim L, Damonte P, Borowsky AD, Qi J, Tepper CG, MacLeod CL, Cardiff RD, Gregg JP (2006) Rapamycin inhibits growth of premalignant and malignant mammary lesions in a mouse model of ductal carcinoma in situ. Clin Cancer Res 12:2613–2621

52. Bonuccelli G, Casimiro MC, Sotgia F, Wang C, Liu M, Katiyar S, Zhou J, Dew E, Capozza F, Daumer KM, Minetti C, Milliman JN, Alpy F, Rio MC, Tomasetto C, Mercier I, Flomenberg N, Frank PG, Pestell RG, Lisanti MP (2009) Caveolin-1 (P132L), a common breast cancer mutation, confers mammary cell invasiveness and defines a novel stem cell/metastasis-associated gene signature. Am J Pathol 174:1650–1662

53. Hennighausen L, Robinson GW (1998) Think globally, act locally: the making of a mouse mammary gland. Genes Dev 12:449–455

54. Freeman ME, Kanyicska B, Lerant A, Nagy G (2000) Prolactin: structure, function, and regulation of secretion. Physiol Rev 80:1523–1631

55. Park DS, Lee H, Riedel C, Hulit J, Scherer PE, Pestell RG, Lisanti MP (2001) Prolactin negatively regulates caveolin-1 gene expression in the mammary gland during lactation, via a Ras-dependent mechanism. J Biol Chem 276:48389–48397

56. Park DS, Lee H, Frank PG, Razani B, Nguyen AV, Parlow AF, Russell RG, Hulit J, Pestell RG, Lisanti MP (2002) Caveolin-1-deficient mice show accelerated mammary gland development during pregnancy, premature lactation, and hyperactivation of the Jak-2/STAT5a signaling cascade. Mol Biol Cell 13:3416–3430

57. Lindeman GJ, Wittlin S, Lada H, Naylor MJ, Santamaria M, Zhang JG, Starr R, Hilton DJ, Alexander WS, Ormandy CJ, Visvader J (2001) SOCS1 deficiency results in accelerated mammary gland development and rescues lactation in prolactin receptor-deficient mice. Genes Dev 15:1631–1636

58. Mercier I, Casimiro MC, Wang C, Rosenberg AL, Quong J, Minkeu A, Allen KG, Danilo C, Sotgia F, Bonuccelli G, Jasmin JF, Xu H, Bosco E, Aronow B, Witkiewicz A, Pestell RG, Knudsen ES, Lisanti MP (2008) Human breast cancer-associated fibroblasts (CAFs) show caveolin-1 downregulation and RB tumor suppressor functional inactivation: implications for the response to hormonal therapy. Cancer Biol Ther 7:1212–1225

59. Sotgia F, Del Galdo F, Casimiro MC, Bonuccelli G, Mercier I, Whitaker-Menezes D, Daumer KM, Zhou J, Wang C, Katiyar S, Xu H, Bosco E, Quong AA, Aronow B, Witkiewicz AK, Minetti C, Frank PG, Jimenez SA, Knudsen ES, Pestell RG, Lisanti MP (2009) Caveolin-1-/-null mammary stromal fibroblasts share characteristics with human breast cancer-associated fibroblasts. Am J Pathol 174:746–761

60. Brotherick I, Robson CN, Browell DA, Shenfine J, White MD, Cunliffe WJ, Shenton BK, Egan M, Webb LA, Lunt LG, Young JR, Higgs MJ (1998) Cytokeratin expression in breast cancer: phenotypic changes associated with disease progression. Cytometry 32:301–308

61. Ronnstrand L, Heldin CH (2001) Mechanisms of platelet-derived growth factor-induced chemotaxis. Int J Cancer 91:757–762

62. Machesky LM (2008) Lamellipodia and filopodia in metastasis and invasion. FEBS Lett 582:2102–2111

63. Sloan EK, Stanley KL, Anderson RL (2004) Caveolin-1 inhibits breast cancer growth and metastasis. Oncogene 23:7893–7897

64. Guy CT, Cardiff RD, Muller WJ (1992) Induction of mammary tumors by expression of polyomavirus middle T oncogene: a transgenic mouse model for metastatic disease. Mol Cell Biol 12:954–961

65. Coussens LM, Werb Z (1996) Matrix metalloproteinases and the development of cancer. Chem Biol 3:895–904

66. Itoh T, Tanioka M, Yoshida H, Yoshioka T, Nishimoto H, Itohara S (1998) Reduced angiogenesis and tumor progression in gelatinase A-deficient mice. Cancer Res 58:1048–1051

67. Itoh T, Tanioka M, Matsuda H, Nishimoto H, Yoshioka T, Suzuki R, Uehira M (1999) Experimental metastasis is suppressed in MMP-9-deficient mice. Clin Exp Metastasis 17:177–181

68. Egeblad M, Werb Z (2002) New functions for the matrix metalloproteinases in cancer progression. Nat Rev Cancer 2:161–174

69. Strongin AY, Collier I, Bannikov G, Marmer BL, Grant GA, Goldberg GI (1995) Mechanism of cell surface activation of 72-kDa type IV collagenase. Isolation of the activated form of the membrane metalloprotease. J Biol Chem 270:5331–5338
70. Puyraimond A, Fridman R, Lemesle M, Arbeille B, Menashi S (2001) MMP-2 colocalizes with caveolae on the surface of endothelial cells. Exp Cell Res 262:28–36
71. Annabi B, Lachambre M, Bousquet-Gagnon N, Page M, Gingras D, Beliveau R (2001) Localization of membrane-type 1 matrix metalloproteinase in caveolae membrane domains. Biochem J 353:547–553
72. Galvez BG, Matias-Roman S, Yanez-Mo M, Vicente-Manzanares M, Sanchez-Madrid F, Arroyo AG (2004) Caveolae are a novel pathway for membrane-type 1 matrix metalloproteinase traffic in human endothelial cells. Mol Biol Cell 15:678–687
73. Engelman JA, Wycoff CC, Yasuhara S, Song KS, Okamoto T, Lisanti MP (1997) Recombinant expression of caveolin-1 in oncogenically transformed cells abrogates anchorage-independent growth. J Biol Chem 272:16374–16381
74. Zundel W, Swiersz LM, Giaccia A (2000) Caveolin 1-mediated regulation of receptor tyrosine kinase-associated phosphatidylinositol 3-kinase activity by ceramide. Mol Cell Biol 20:1507–1514
75. Liu J, Lee P, Galbiati F, Kitsis RN, Lisanti MP (2001) Caveolin-1 expression sensitizes fibroblastic and epithelial cells to apoptotic stimulation. Am J Physiol Cell Physiol 280:C823–C835
76. Li L, Yang G, Ebara S, Satoh T, Nasu Y, Timme TL, Ren C, Wang J, Tahir SA, Thompson TC (2001) Caveolin-1 mediates testosterone-stimulated survival/clonal growth and promotes metastatic activities in prostate cancer cells. Cancer Res 61:4386–4392
77. Nasu Y, Timme TL, Yang G, Bangma CH, Li L, Ren C, Park SH, DeLeon M, Wang J, Thompson TC (1998) Suppression of caveolin expression induces androgen sensitivity in metastatic androgen-insensitive mouse prostate cancer cells. Nat Med 4:1062–1064
78. Pavlides S, Whitaker-Menezes D, Castello-Cros R, Flomenberg N, Witkiewicz AK, Frank PG, Casimiro MC, Wang C, Fortina P, Addya S, Pestell RG, Martinez-Outschoorn UE, Sotgia F, Lisanti MP (2009) The reverse Warburg effect: aerobic glycolysis in cancer associated fibroblasts and the tumor stroma. Cell Cycle 8:3984–4001
79. Martinez-Outschoorn UE, Balliet RM, Rivadeneira DB, Chiavarina B, Pavlides S, Wang C, Whitaker-Menezes D, Daumer KM, Lin Z, Witkiewicz AK, Flomenberg N, Howell A, Pestell RG, Knudsen ES, Sotgia F, Lisanti MP (2010) Oxidative stress in cancer associated fibroblasts drives tumor-stroma co-evolution: a new paradigm for understanding tumor metabolism, the field effect and genomic instability in cancer cells. Cell Cycle 9:3256–3276
80. Martinez-Outschoorn UE, Trimmer C, Lin Z, Whitaker-Menezes D, Chiavarina B, Zhou J, Wang C, Pavlides S, Martinez-Cantarin MP, Capozza F, Witkiewicz AK, Flomenberg N, Howell A, Pestell RG, Caro J, Lisanti MP, Sotgia F (2010) Autophagy in cancer associated fibroblasts promotes tumor cell survival: role of hypoxia, HIF1 induction and NFkappaB activation in the tumor stromal microenvironment. Cell Cycle 9:3515–3533
81. Bonuccelli G, Tsirigos A, Whitaker-Menezes D, Pavlides S, Pestell RG, Chiavarina B, Frank PG, Flomenberg N, Howell A, Martinez-Outschoorn UE, Sotgia F, Lisanti MP (2010) Ketones and lactate "fuel" tumor growth and metastasis: evidence that epithelial cancer cells use oxidative mitochondrial metabolism. Cell Cycle 9:3506–3514
82. Pavlides S, Tsirigos A, Migneco G, Whitaker-Menezes D, Chiavarina B, Flomenberg N, Frank PG, Casimiro MC, Wang C, Pestell RG, Martinez-Outschoorn UE, Howell A, Sotgia F, Lisanti MP (2010) The autophagic tumor stroma model of cancer: role of oxidative stress and ketone production in fueling tumor cell metabolism. Cell Cycle 9:3485–3505
83. Witkiewicz AK, Dasgupta A, Sotgia F, Mercier I, Pestell RG, Sabel M, Kleer CG, Brody JR, Lisanti MP (2009) An absence of stromal caveolin-1 expression predicts early tumor recurrence and poor clinical outcome in human breast cancers. Am J Pathol 174:2023–2034
84. Pavlides S, Tsirigos A, Vera I, Flomenberg N, Frank PG, Casimiro MC, Wang C, Fortina P, Addya S, Pestell RG, Martinez-Outschoorn UE, Sotgia F, Lisanti MP (2010) Loss of stromal caveolin-1 leads to oxidative stress, mimics hypoxia and drives inflammation in the tumor microenvironment, conferring the "reverse Warburg effect": a transcriptional informatics analysis with validation. Cell Cycle 9:2201–2219

85. Lisanti MP, Martinez-Outschoorn UE, Chiavarina B, Pavlides S, Whitaker-Menezes D, Tsirigos A, Witkiewicz A, Lin Z, Balliet R, Howell A, Sotgia F (2010) Understanding the "lethal" drivers of tumor-stroma co-evolution: emerging role(s) for hypoxia, oxidative stress and autophagy/mitophagy in the tumor micro-environment. Cancer Biol Ther 10:537–542
86. Chiavarina B, Whitaker-Menezes D, Migneco G, Martinez-Outschoorn UE, Pavlides S, Howell A, Tanowitz HB, Casimiro MC, Wang C, Pestell RG, Grieshaber P, Caro J, Sotgia F, Lisanti MP (2010) HIF1-alpha functions as a tumor promoter in cancer associated fibroblasts, and as a tumor suppressor in breast cancer cells: autophagy drives compartment-specific oncogenesis. Cell Cycle 9:3534–3551
87. Nakamura Y, Yasuoka H, Tsujimoto M, Yoshidome K, Nakahara M, Nakao K, Nakamura M, Kakudo K (2006) Nitric oxide in breast cancer: induction of vascular endothelial growth factor-C and correlation with metastasis and poor prognosis. Clin Cancer Res 12:1201–1207
88. Witkiewicz AK, Casimiro MC, Dasgupta A, Mercier I, Wang C, Bonuccelli G, Jasmin JF, Frank PG, Pestell RG, Kleer CG, Sotgia F, Lisanti MP (2009) Towards a new "stromal-based" classification system for human breast cancer prognosis and therapy. Cell Cycle 8:1654–1658
89. Witkiewicz AK, Dasgupta A, Nguyen KH, Liu C, Kovatich AJ, Schwartz GF, Pestell RG, Sotgia F, Rui H, Lisanti MP (2009) Stromal caveolin-1 levels predict early DCIS progression to invasive breast cancer. Cancer Biol Ther 8:1071–1079
90. Di Vizio D, Morello M, Sotgia F, Pestell RG, Freeman MR, Lisanti MP (2009) An absence of stromal caveolin-1 is associated with advanced prostate cancer, metastatic disease and epithelial Akt activation. Cell Cycle 8:2420–2424
91. Migneco G, Whitaker-Menezes D, Chiavarina B, Castello-Cros R, Pavlides S, Pestell RG, Fatatis A, Flomenberg N, Tsirigos A, Howell A, Martinez-Outschoorn UE, Sotgia F, Lisanti MP (2010) Glycolytic cancer associated fibroblasts promote breast cancer tumor growth, without a measurable increase in angiogenesis: evidence for stromal-epithelial metabolic coupling. Cell Cycle 9:2412–2422
92. Pennacchietti S, Michieli P, Galluzzo M, Mazzone M, Giordano S, Comoglio PM (2003) Hypoxia promotes invasive growth by transcriptional activation of the met protooncogene. Cancer Cell 3:347–361
93. Steeg PS (2003) Angiogenesis inhibitors: motivators of metastasis? Nat Med 9:822–823
94. Grepin R, Pages G (2010) Molecular mechanisms of resistance to tumour anti-angiogenic strategies. J Oncol 2010:835680

Chapter 8
Caveolin-1 and Cancer-Associated Stromal Fibroblasts

Isabelle Mercier and Michael P. Lisanti

The Cancer Stroma: An Unrelenting Wounding Process

Tumors are a complex array of different cell types that are far from isolated, but rather intertwined with each other, such as epithelial, stromal and inflammatory cells, as well as endothelial cells that constitute the vessels which supply nutrients and oxygen to tumors. To completely eradicate cancer, every component of a tumor needs to be carefully studied, both individually and as a total entity to better comprehend cancer initiation, progression, response to chemotherapy, and clinical prognosis. Interestingly, pathologists were the first to detect fibroblasts in the tumor stroma, simply describing them as myofibroblasts (a hybrid cell type that is somewhere between a fibroblast and a smooth muscle cell). Cancer-associated fibroblast (CAFs) can sometimes constitute up to 50–70% of the tumor, making these cells the most abundant in the cancer stroma and the most well-studied [5].

Following the discovery of CAFs, researchers began to compare their characteristics with those of fibroblasts associated with wound healing. In fact, shortly following an injury, the repair process begins by the transformation and differentiation of fibroblasts into contractile myofibroblast cells to promote the narrowing of a wound. This process is accompanied by a massive synthesis of extracellular matrix (ECM) proteins that will lay down a structural scaffolding network, to allow the movement of fibroblasts and attract epithelial cells to cover the wound. These events are driven by a local release of cytokines and inflammatory intermediaries, and by the activated fibroblasts themselves [6, 7]. Surprisingly, CAFs share similar expression of "wound healing" mesenchymal proteins, such as alpha-smooth muscle actin (α-SMA), vimentin, smooth muscle myosin, tenascin, desmin, calponin, and they lack expression of epithelial and endothelial markers, such as cytokeratin and CD31,

I. Mercier (✉) • M.P. Lisanti (✉)
Department of Stem Cell Biology & Regenerative Medicine, Thomas Jefferson University,
Philadelphia, PA, USA
e-mail: isabelle.mercier@jefferson.edu; mlisanti@KimmelCancerCenter.org

I. Mercier et al. (eds.), *Caveolins in Cancer Pathogenesis, Prevention and Therapy*,
Current Cancer Research, DOI 10.1007/978-1-4614-1001-0_8,
© Springer Science+Business Media, LLC 2012

respectively [8–11]. Consequently, the understanding of the role of CAFs was greatly accelerated by the previous characterization and understanding of wound healing fibroblasts [12]. In fact, only a few known differences exist between wound healing and CAFs, the main one involving apoptosis. Indeed, activated fibroblasts implicated in acute repair undergo spontaneous apoptosis once the healing process is completed, while distinctively, CAFs do not participate in programmed cells death and continue to actively proliferate and secrete growth factors. Thus, it was anticipated that a wound healing stroma would be more susceptible to tumor development and would constitute a more suitable "soil" than a normal non-activated; stroma. As such, Dingemans et al. demonstrated that cancer cells transplanted into developing subcutaneous granulation tissue formed more invasive tumors than those transplanted in undisturbed tissue [13]. These experiments dramatically validated the striking similarities between wound healing and cancer-associated stroma, and allowed a clearer understanding of the contribution of fibroblasts to tumor growth and invasiveness.

CAFs: Catalysts for Tumor Growth

The main characteristic of a cancer-associated stroma is a noticeable desmoplasia, which results from hyperplasic fibroblasts that produce the excessive secretion of ECM proteins, such as collagen around the tumor. An example of a reactive breast tumor stroma is shown in Fig. 8.1a (left panel), which depicts an extensive collagen network with the presence of increased number of CAFs surrounding the epithelial tumor cells [14]. The increased number of fibroblasts in the cancer stroma is thought to arise from increased proliferation. We recently validated this hypothesis by isolating primary fibroblast cultures from freshly excised breast tumors and by measuring their cell cycle activity. As such, we demonstrated that CAFs from human breast tumors were more elongated and had a spindle shape when compared with normal fibroblasts (NFs) isolated from adjacent benign breast tissue of the same patient (Fig. 8.1a; left panel). In addition, these mammary CAFs showed increased BrdU incorporation, a thymide analogue that reflects active DNA synthesis (Fig. 8.1a; right panel) [14].

Several studies have now demonstrated that CAFs represent a direct tumor-promoting force, as shown by co-culture and tissue recombination experiments, as they can drive the progression of "benign" cells to a frank tumorigenic phenotype. For example, the combination of normal prostatic epithelial cells with CAFs isolated from prostate tumors induced the formation of PIN (prostatic intraepithelial neoplasia)-like lesions. More interestingly, when the same experiment was repeated with the combination of immortalized prostatic epithelial cells and CAFs, the tumors that developed were 500-fold bigger than the graft that contained the same epithelial cells with NFs [15]. More precisely, the addition of CAFs altered the cell morphology, decreased the number of apoptotic cells, and increased the proliferation rate of prostatic epithelial cells [15]. Similar results were obtained when epithelial cells from the

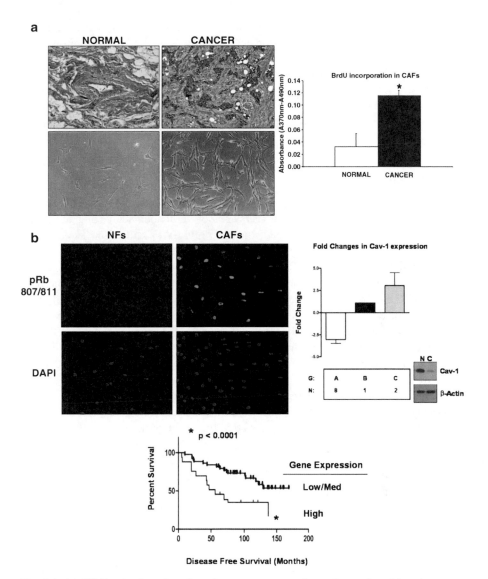

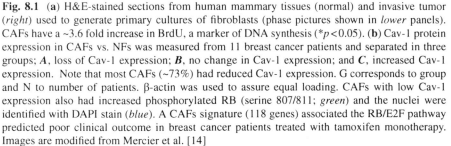

Fig. 8.1 (a) H&E-stained sections from human mammary tissues (normal) and invasive tumor (*right*) used to generate primary cultures of fibroblasts (phase pictures shown in *lower* panels). CAFs have a ~3.6 fold increase in BrdU, a marker of DNA synthesis (*$p < 0.05$). (b) Cav-1 protein expression in CAFs vs. NFs was measured from 11 breast cancer patients and separated in three groups; *A*, loss of Cav-1 expression; *B*, no change in Cav-1 expression; and *C*, increased Cav-1 expression. Note that most CAFs (~73%) had reduced Cav-1 expression. G corresponds to group and N to number of patients. β-actin was used to assure equal loading. CAFs with low Cav-1 expression also had increased phosphorylated RB (serine 807/811; *green*) and the nuclei were identified with DAPI stain (*blue*). A CAFs signature (118 genes) associated the RB/E2F pathway predicted poor clinical outcome in breast cancer patients treated with tamoxifen monotherapy. Images are modified from Mercier et al. [14]

pancreas were exposed to the culture media of pancreatic CAFs, showing increased proliferation and exaggerated migration and invasion potential [16]. Barcellos-Hoff et al. have shown that cleared mouse mammary fat pads (in which the epithelial component has been removed) can develop larger tumors following ionizing irradiation, a well-described mutagen [17]. These findings separated the epithelial vs. stromal components of the fat pad, and suggested that exposure of the stroma to known mutagens could be sufficient to promote and accelerate tumor formation in vivo.

The Source and Origin of CAFs

Despite the discovery of CAFs several years ago now, both their source and origin still remain ambiguous and poorly defined. Interestingly, CAFs can differ according to tumor type, thus introducing additional complexity in understanding the role of this cell type in tumor pathogenesis [18]. For example, breast and pancreatic CAFs can be divided in two main subtypes; those that are positive for the fibroblast-specific protein-1 (FSP1) and negative for the neuron-glial antigen-2 (NG2), αSMA, and PDGF β-receptor and, conversely, those that are FSP1-negative while positive for NG2, αSMA, and PDGF β-receptor [19]. More subgroups of CAFs may exist that still have yet to be characterized and will, thus, have to be attentively studied to understand their contribution to tumor pathogenesis and progression. When originally discovered, locally-residing NFs were believed to be the primary precursors of activated CAFs. Indeed, local NFs undergo a transformation process during cancer that leads to increased contractility, enhanced proliferative index, and a sustained increase in ECM production [4]. Although extensively debated, the in situ origin of CAFs has been confirmed in vitro. Indeed, some studies have established that NFs exposed to CAFs in co-culture was sufficient to convert them into α-SMA-expressing myofibroblasts [20, 21]. In addition, treatment with TGFβ (transforming growth factor beta) was later shown to induce the production of collagen and α-SMA in cultured NFs [22].

In addition to local residing NFs, other sources are thought to serve as precursors of CAFs. For example, mesenchymal bone-marrow-derived cells have also been established as precursors of CAFs, as demonstrated by the transplantation of bone marrow cells tagged with a green fluorescent protein (GFP), in a murine model of pancreatic cancer [23, 24]. In addition, the exposure of human bone marrow-derived mesenchymal stem cells to tumor cell-derived conditioned media resulted in the acquisition of CAFs-like properties, such as the expression of α-SMA and FSP1 [25]. Lastly, both epithelial and endothelial cells have also been shown to serve as "potential precursors" of CAFs, as they can undergo a mesenchymal transition or trans-differentiation, as previously published [26, 27]. Together, these recent observations suggest that both the subtypes, as well as the origin of activated tumor fibroblasts, could be important in understanding tumor heterogeneity and account for the different responses of patients to hormonal and chemotherapeutic agents. Further studies are warranted to fully comprehend the complexity of these multifaceted cells and their exact role(s) in cancer pathogenesis.

CAFs Promote Tumor Angiogenesis

Angiogenesis, the development of new capillaries from pre-existing vessels, is induced in important physiological processes such as embryogenesis and wound repair, as well as the menstrual cycle [28]. Angiogenic responses can either be helpful or detrimental, depending on the tissue and the type of pathology. Although the formation of collaterals as a result of angiogenesis is beneficial following ischemic cardiovascular diseases, angiogenesis that surrounds tumor growth is detrimental to survival of the organism, since it increases the supply of nutrients and oxygen and supports cancer growth. The epithelial tumor cells can secrete factors that stimulate neovascularization, thus directly sustaining their own growth and survival. Several studies have demonstrated that blockade of angiogenesis-related signaling pathway(s) causes tumors to shrink considerably due to starvation and subsequent necrosis [29]. While epithelial cells have been considered the main cell type involved in tumor-associated angiogenesis, there is new evidence that stromal cells, more specifically CAFs, can actively regulate this process. Some studies have shown that human breast CAFs can induce tumor growth significantly more than NFs isolated from the same patient and support increased vascularization, suggestive of angiogenesis [30]. More interestingly, CAFs were shown to promote neovascularization through their ability to recruit and mobilize endothelial progenitor cells to the tumor mass, and facilitating their differentiation into vascular endothelial cells [30]. The angiogenesis-promoting feature of CAFs could also play an important role in other types of cancers, such as pancreatic cancer [31]. Together, these observations suggest that stromal cells, specifically CAFs, could become effective targets for inhibiting tumor growth and angiogenesis in patients.

Caveolin-1 (Cav-1) and the Cancer Stroma

Until recently, the role of caveolin proteins in the stroma of cancer patients has remained completely unknown. Caveolae are small invaginations of the cell membrane that take part in important biological processes, such as endocytosis, the uptake of viruses and bacteria, as well as bringing in proximity important signaling molecules, thus, facilitating their interactions with one another. Caveolin-1 (Cav-1) is an important structural protein that is responsible for the formation and maintenance of caveolae architecture and is mainly expressed in endothelial, epithelial, and myo-epithelial cells as well as fibroblasts, adipocytes, and type I pneumocytes [32]. Cav-1 is versatile as it can behave as a tumor suppressor or a tumor promoter depending on the tissue origin [33]. In breast tissue, Cav-1 seems to consistently behave as a tumor suppressor. In accordance, total genetic ablation of Cav-1 (Cav-1 KO) accelerates the appearance of dysplastic foci and facilitates the formation of mammary tumors when interbred with another mouse model of carcinogenesis, such as mouse mammary tumor virus LTR-driven polyoma middle T antigen (MMTV-PyMT) mice. In cell culture experiments, NIH3T3 fibroblasts transformed with a variety of well-characterized oncogenes, such as H-Ras (G12V) and v-Abl, caused a significant decrease in the endogenous levels of Cav-1 [34]. Mechanistically, Cav-1 expression has been shown to inhibit cell growth by inducing a G0/G1 cell cycle arrest [35, 36].

Thus, it remained unknown whether Cav-1 can behave as an endogenous regulator of mammary stromal fibroblast (MSF) growth and if a decrease in Cav-1 could result in increased proliferation and be associated with a poor clinical prognosis in patients. To directly test this hypothesis, isolated CAFs from freshly excised breast tumors from women with invasive breast cancer were cultured. Fibroblasts from normal breast tissue were isolated from the same patient and used as controls throughout the experiments [14]. When left to grow for 72 h in culture, CAFs had an elongated and spindled-shape morphology and incorporated ~3.6-fold more BrdU than NFs, confirming that CAFs populations had increased DNA synthesis, when compared with fibroblasts surrounding normal breast tissue (Fig. 8.1a; right panel). These CAFs had decreased levels of the retinoblastoma (RB) protein, a potent tumor suppressor, as reflected by an increase in its inactivating phosphorylations at serines 807 and 811 when compared to NFs (Fig. 8.1b; left panel). These results suggest that CAFs can proliferate faster through a RB-dependent pathway. More interestingly, almost 73% (8/11) of patients with invasive breast cancer showed a significant decrease in Cav-1 protein levels in their proliferative CAFs, when compared with fibroblasts surrounding the normal breast tissue (Fig. 8.1b; right panel) [14]. To gain further mechanistic insight on the role of Cav-1 in stromal cells, we performed genome-wide transcriptional profiling on breast CAFs (isolated from three patients with decreased Cav-1 levels) and matching NFs to identify a CAF-specific gene signature. Remarkably, this CAF-related gene signature (118 up-regulated transcripts) closely associated with a previously described tamoxifen-resistance transcriptional "fingerprint" [14]. More precisely, CAFs with decreased Cav-1 levels had a similar gene profile as patients with a decrease in recurrence-free survival following tamoxifen mono-therapy (Fig. 8.1b; lower panel) [14]. Mechanistically, we believe that Cav-1 levels in CAFs are regulated post-transcriptionally, as demonstrated by a lack of decrease in Cav-1 mRNA levels in human breast CAFs. Future studies will be required to confirm this hypothesis, both in vitro and in vivo.

A Cav-1 Mimetic Peptide Inhibits the Growth of Human CAFs: A Novel Stromal Therapeutic Approach

In addition to sharing a gene signature that predicts the response of breast cancer patients to tamoxifen, comparative analysis of human breast CAFs (with low Cav-1 expression) resulted in a gene expression signature that was closely associated with the RB pathway (Table 8.1) [14]. Surprisingly, 44 genes among the total 118 genes up-regulated were part of an RB/E2F gene signature associated with the RB pathway. These findings are consistent with increased levels of phosphorylated RB found in CAFs. Indeed, when RB is hypo-phosphorylated, it can bind E2F family transcription factors, and subsequently suppress the transcription of genes necessary for cell-cycle

Table 8.1 Breast CAFs RB/E2F-Associated Gene Signature (44 up-regulated genes).

ANLN	Anillin, actin binding protein (scraps homolog, Drosophila)
AURKA	Aurora kinase A
BIRC5	Baculoviral IAP repeat-containing 5 (survivin)
BLM	Bloom syndrome
BRCA1	Breast cancer 1, early onset
BUB1	BUB1 budding uninhibited by benzimidazoles 1 homolog (yeast)
CCNB2	Cyclin B2
CCNF	Cyclin F
CDC2	Cell division cycle 2, G1 to S and G2 to M
CDC20	CDC20 cell division cycle 20 homolog (*Saccharomyces cerevisiae*)
CDC45L	CDC45 cell division cycle 45-like (*S. cerevisiae*)
CDCA3	Cell division cycle associated 3
CDCA5	Cell division cycle associated 5
CDCA8	Cell division cycle associated 8
CENPA	Centromere protein A
FANCD2	Fanconi anemia, complementation group D2
FOXM1	Forkhead box M1
GTSE1	G-2 and S-phase expressed 1
KIF11	Kinesin family member 11
KIF20A	Kinesin family member 20A
KIF23	Kinesin family member 23
KIF2C	Kinesin family member 2C
KIF4A	Kinesin family member 4A
MAD2L1	MAD2 mitotic arrest deficient-like 1 (yeast)
MCM10	MCM10 minichromosome maintenance deficient 10 (*S. cerevisiae*)
MCM2	MCM2 minichromosome maintenance deficient 2, mitotin (*S. cerevisiae*)
MCM5	MCM5 minichromosome maintenance deficient 5, cell division cycle 46 (*S. cerevisiae*)
MKI67	Antigen identified by monoclonal antibody Ki-67
NEK2	NIMA (never in mitosis gene a)-related kinase 2
NUSAP1	Nucleolar and spindle associated protein 1
PLK1	Polo-like kinase 1 (Drosophila)
PRC1	Protein regulator of cytokinesis 1
PRIM1	Primase, polypeptide 1, 49 kDa
PTTG1	Pituitary tumor-transforming 1
RAD51AP1	RAD51 associated protein 1
RAD54L	RAD54-like (*S. cerevisiae*)
RRM2	Ribonucleotide reductase M2 polypeptide
STMN1	Stathmin 1/oncoprotein 18
TCF19	Transcription factor 19 (SC1)
TK1	Thymidine kinase 1, soluble
TOP2A	Topoisomerase (DNA) II alpha 170 kDa
TRIP13	Thyroid hormone receptor interactor 13
TTK	TTK protein kinase
TYMS	Thymidylate synthetase

progression [37]. To further validate this RB-dependent signature, we analyzed the expression of downstream targets of hyper-phosphorylated RB, such as minichromosome maintenance protein (MCM7) and proliferating cell nuclear antigen (PCNA), two important replication factors. Consistent with RB inactivation, MCM7 and PCNA protein expressions were significantly induced in the nucleus of CAFs, when compared with NFs [14].

To demonstrate a direct functional role for Cav-1 on RB signaling in the stroma, CAFs were treated with a cell-permeable Cav-1 mimetic peptide, corresponding to its active scaffolding domain [14]. This peptide was previously shown to inhibit tumor progression, proliferation, and inflammation in mice [38, 39]. As predicted, the treatment of CAFs with a Cav-1 mimetic peptide reduced DNA synthesis, as shown by BrdU incorporation and significantly inhibited RB phosphorylation, as well as PCNA levels (Fig. 8.2a) [14]. These results are mechanistically important as they show that a decrease in Cav-1 levels in CAFs could play an important role in regulating their proliferation and the pathogenesis of breast cancer, through a RB-dependent pathway. Understanding the functional role of Cav-1 in breast CAFs could lead to the development of new stromal-targeted therapies to treat breast cancer patients.

Stromal Cav-1 as a New Predictor of Disease Outcome in Cancer Patients

Typically, tumor staging and epithelial expression of estrogen receptor (ER), progesterone receptor (PR), and human epidermal growth factor receptor 2 (HER2) have been used to stratify breast cancer patients, assign appropriate treatment, and predict survival [40]. However, these parameters are currently insufficient for predicting resistance to chemotherapy and patient outcome. The lack of accuracy in predicting patient outcome could be explained by the resistance to incorporate stromal-specific markers in the current classification. Indeed, the absence of stromal biomarkers in the existing breast cancer classification is surprising; especially with all the available data that suggest the dynamic contribution of the tumor microenvironment to cancer pathogenesis. As previously mentioned, we demonstrated that primary cultures of human breast CAFs that have a decrease in Cav-1 levels demonstrate an inactivated form of RB (a potent tumor suppressor) and a molecular gene signature that is associated with tamoxifen-resistance and poor clinical outcome [14]. As such, we and others have recently examined the prognostic significance of stromal Cav-1 in human breast cancers [41, 42]. The stromal Cav-1 levels were assessed in paraffin-embedded human breast tumors using tissue microarrays (TMAs), as a mean to predict clinical outcome and response to chemotherapy. Our analysis showed that failure to express the Cav-1 protein in the stroma of human breast tumors correlated with early disease recurrence, lymph node metastasis, tamoxifen-resistance, as well as advanced tumor and nodal staging (Fig. 8.2b) [41]. More specifically,

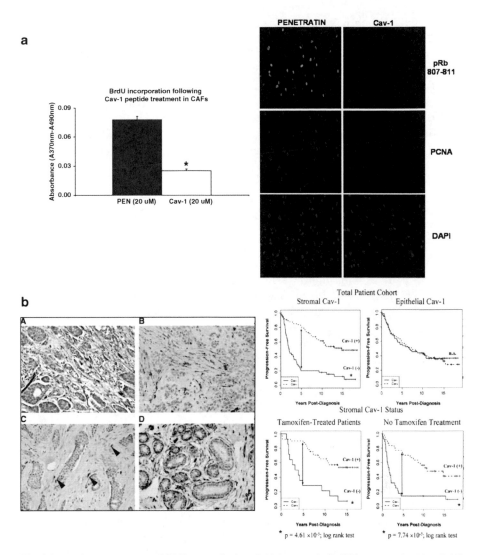

Fig. 8.2 (a) Cav-1 treatment of CAFs caused a threefold decrease in BrdU incorporation (*$p < 0.05$) and inhibited the phosphorylation of RB (S807/811; *green*) and PCNA (*red*) as shown by immunofluorescence compared to penetratrin alone (*right side*; *upper* panels). DAPI staining (*blue*) shows the nuclei (images were taken at 20x). (**b**) Human breast tumor microarrays were immunostained with an antibody directed against Cav-1. Panels **A** and **B** show Cav-1 expression in the stroma of invasive ductal carcinomas. Panel **C** and **D** show an absence of Cav-1 in the neoplastic stroma and normal human breast tissue (TDLUs; terminal ductal lobular units), arrowheads indicate endothelial cells. As reflected by Kaplan-Meier curves of progression-free survival, only stromal Cav-1 is a predictor of clinical outcome ($p = 1.77 \times 10^{-9}$, log-rank test) and can also predict the outcome in tamoxifen-treated ($p = 14.61 \times 10^{-5}$) and non-treated patients ($p = 7.74 \times 10^{-5}$). A 5-year progression free survival is indicated by an arrow. Images are modified from Mercier et al. [14] and Witkiewicz et al. [41]

patients with lymph node involvement showed the largest differences in 5-year progression-free survival, with an 80% chance of survival if they expressed Cav-1 in their tumor stroma. Surprisingly, the levels of epithelial Cav-1 had no clinical value compared to stromal Cav-1 (Fig. 8.2b). Ductal carcinomas in situ (DCIS) is a pre-invasive lesion that constitutes more than 30% of breast carcinomas diagnosed in the United States. Several studies suggest that DCIS lesions are precursors to invasive breast cancer and patients often receive tamoxifen or radiation therapy. However, some DCIS lesions can remain benign and do not require further treatment [43]. We recently demonstrated that stromal Cav-1 levels can be used as a novel biomarker to accurately predict which DCIS patient will progress to invasive breast cancer [44]. Using a cohort of 56 ER-positive breast cancer patients, we aimed to determine the association of stromal Cav-1 levels with DCIS recurrence and/or progression to invasive breast cancer. In our cohort, the majority of patients (90%) that evolved to invasive breast cancer had reduced or absent levels of Cav-1. This absence of Cav-1 correlated with accelerated recurrence and early progression to invasive breast cancer. Surprisingly, 97% of ER (+) DCIS patients with high levels of stromal Cav-1 remained free of invasive disease recurrence [44]. Taken together, these results suggest that Cav-1 could become an important predictive tool and a new biomarker for directing the treatment of ER (+) DCIS patients.

In addition, our recent work suggests that the predictive value of stromal Cav-1 levels is not restricted to breast cancer. In fact, our results demonstrate a novel association of stromal Cav-1 levels with prostate cancer progression. As expected, patients with benign prostate hypertrophy (BPH) have abundant levels of stromal Cav-1, while patients with primary prostate cancer show decreased levels of Cav-1 expression in their stromal compartment, which correlate with a high Gleason's score and poor prognosis [45]. As one would expect, all metastases that were isolated from the bones or lymph nodes were completely depleted of Cav-1 in their stromal compartment. These results could especially be important in the context of advanced prostate cancer and hormone-refractory disease. Since prostate growth and function require androgen actions through the androgen receptor (AR), most prostate cancers are androgen-dependent and rely on the presence of testosterone for growth and progression. As a result of this reliance on androgen, the current most effective treatment for prostate cancer is androgen-deprivation therapy in the form of pharmacological or surgical castration that inhibits AR-dependent proliferation [46]. Unfortunately, most patients under these regimens will inevitably relapse with a more aggressive form of the cancer that has been termed hormone refractory prostate cancer (HRPC) [47]. From this point, the tumors become unresponsive to further hormonal manipulation and respond poorly to chemotherapy, decreasing a patient's chance for survival. Thus, new biomarkers that could predict early on which patients will progress toward HRPC status are desperately needed and stromal Cav-1 could meet these needs. Understanding the role of Cav-1 in prostate tumor stroma could also open new therapeutic avenues that could help in the effective treatment of prostate cancer.

Cav-1 Knockout (Cav-1 KO) Mice: A New Preclinical Model to Study the Role of Stromal Cav-1 in Cancer Pathogenesis and Progression

Experiments using a mouse model with deleted Cav-1 on both alleles (Cav-1 KO) were undertaken to assess the functional role of stromal Cav-1 in the mammary gland. Mouse mammary fat pads were modified to create an epithelia-free host that can be further used to study specifically the effects of the stroma on tumor growth. Using this technique, normal epithelia and mammary tumor pieces were transplanted in the epithelia-free stroma of mice lacking Cav-1 and compared with that of wild type mice. Interestingly, in these experiments, Cav-1 KO mice mammary stroma was shown to behave as a potent catalyst for hyperplasia and full blown tumorigenesis [48]. This was the first in vivo study demonstrating that Cav-1 expression confers protection against proliferation in the stromal compartment and suggested that Cav-1 KO mice could be used to study the mammary stroma and serve as a preclinical model to test new stromal therapies. In addition, we recently showed that Cav-1 KO mice can develop high-grade DCIS-like lesions with micro-invasion and amplified mammary stromal angiogenesis, following estrogen treatment [49]. We believe that estrogen-induced DCIS formation is a stromal phenomenon due to the lack of Cav-1 expression in the stromal compartment. We predict that if treated with estrogen for a longer time point (6–12 months), these DCIS lesions could develop into full blown invasive lesions. This would suggest that DCIS patients with decreased stromal Cav-1 would be more sensitive to the proliferative effects of estrogen and could be more prone to develop fully invasive tumors, compared with those with elevated Cav-1. In addition, the lack of improvement in survival of some ER-positive DCIS patients, following tamoxifen treatment, could be explained by the lack of Cav-1 in their tumor stroma. Accordingly, our Cav-1 KO DCIS mouse model shows a massive up-regulation of B23/nucleophosmin (a known marker of tamoxifen-resistance) suggesting that a lack of Cav-1 in the mammary fat pad could make these mice more sensitive to the proliferative effects of estrogen, while inducing tamoxifen resistance [49]. Thus, a clinical assessment of Cav-1 stromal status in estrogen-positive DCIS patients could become a new diagnostic tool.

Interestingly, we recently discovered that MSFs that originate from Cav-1 KO mice share several characteristics with our previously characterized human CAFs population [50]. Indeed, Cav-1 KO MSFs demonstrated a myofibroblast-like morphology, as demonstrated through the increased expression of muscle-related genes such as SMA, aniline, merosin, myosin, and tropomyosin [50]. In agreement with the activation of TGF-β/Smad signaling driving the transformation of fibroblasts into myofibroblasts, our DNA microarray and RT-PCR results demonstrated that Cav-1 KO MSFs showed increased levels of TGF-β/Smad-responsive genes such as SMA, collagen I, interleukin-11, TGF-β ligand(s), and connective tissue growth factor (CTGF) [50]. Consistent with a myofibroblastic phenotype, Cav-1 KO MSFs showed intense F-actin stress fibers, as well as increased collagen I secretion, as shown by immunofluorescence studies. More importantly, MSFs isolated from Cav-1 KO mice demonstrated a nearly identical RB/E2F gene signature as the one previously shown in human breast CAFs [50]. These observations were associated with RB inactivation in Cav-1 KO MSFs, as assessed by its hyper-phosphorylation by immunofluorescence analysis. Interestingly, MSFs lacking Cav-1 expression secreted more pro-proliferative and pro-angiogenic growth factors into their culture media, affecting the neighbor epithelial cells through paracrine mechanisms. In fact, our results show that when primary WT mammary epithelial cells are treated with the conditioned media from Cav-1 KO MSFs, they undergo an epithelial–mesenchymal transition (EMT), with enhanced fibroblast-like morphology, as well as increased staining of SMA, an EMT marker [50]. Mechanistically, these results are consistent with the paracrine effects that human CAFs are thought to have on adjacent cancer epithelial cells. These results could explain why cancer patients with lower stromal Cav-1 levels in their tumor fibroblasts have a worse clinical prognosis.

Summary

In conclusion, primary cultures of CAFs isolated from human breast cancers show reduced Cav-1 protein levels and a RB/E2F gene signature that associates with resistance to tamoxifen, when compared to matching NFs. When rescued with exogenous Cav-1 via a cell-permeable mimetic peptide, these CAFs undergo growth inhibition and de-phosphorylation of RB, with a decrease in PCNA levels, demonstrating the potential therapeutic of stromal Cav-1 replacement therapy. When a cohort of breast cancer patients was studied, decreased stromal Cav-1 levels correlated with poor clinical outcome and even predicted which DCIS patient would progress to invasive breast cancer. Using Cav-1 KO mice as a preclinical model, a loss of Cav-1 was shown to contribute to accelerated tumor growth, increased angiogenesis, and even estrogen hyper-sensitivity that can, for the most part, be attributed to a lack of Cav-1 expression in the stroma. More studies are required to dissect the signaling mechanism(s) activated by a lack of Cav-1 in the stroma and the downstream pathways affected and the potential of a stromal-specific Cav-1 therapy. Thus, new personalized therapies could be developed to effectively treat high risk cancer patients that lack stromal Cav-1, by targeting the tumor stromal microenvironment.

References

1. Dunning AM et al (1999) A systematic review of genetic polymorphisms and breast cancer risk. Cancer Epidemiol Biomarkers Prev 8:843–854
2. Park YH et al (2010) A risk stratification by hormonal receptors (ER, PgR) and HER-2 status in small (< or = 1 cm) invasive breast cancer: who might be possible candidates for adjuvant treatment? Breast Cancer Res Treat 119:653–661
3. Ryan BM et al (2006) Survivin expression in breast cancer predicts clinical outcome and is associated with HER2, VEGF, urokinase plasminogen activator and PAI-1. Ann Oncol 17:597–604
4. Ostman A, Augsten M (2009) Cancer-associated fibroblasts and tumor growth – bystanders turning into key players. Curr Opin Genet Dev 19:67–73
5. Desmouliere A, Guyot C, Gabbiani G (2004) The stroma reaction myofibroblast: a key player in the control of tumor cell behavior. Int J Dev Biol 48:509–517
6. Eyden B (2008) The myofibroblast: phenotypic characterization as a prerequisite to understanding its functions in translational medicine. J Cell Mol Med 12:22–37
7. De Wever O, Mareel M (2003) Role of tissue stroma in cancer cell invasion. J Pathol 200:429–447
8. van den Hooff A (1988) Stromal involvement in malignant growth. Adv Cancer Res 50:159–196
9. Mackie EJ et al (1987) Tenascin is a stromal marker for epithelial malignancy in the mammary gland. Proc Natl Acad Sci USA 84:4621–4625
10. Sappino AP, Skalli O, Jackson B, Schurch W, Gabbiani G (1988) Smooth-muscle differentiation in stromal cells of malignant and non-malignant breast tissues. Int J Cancer 41:707–712
11. Gonda TA, Varro A, Wang TC, Tycko B (2010) Molecular biology of cancer-associated fibroblasts: can these cells be targeted in anti-cancer therapy? Semin Cell Dev Biol 21:2–10
12. Dvorak HF (1986) Tumors: wounds that do not heal Similarities between tumor stroma generation and wound healing. N Engl J Med 315:1650–1659
13. Dingemans KP, Zeeman-Boeschoten IM, Keep RF, Das PK (1993) Transplantation of colon carcinoma into granulation tissue induces an invasive morphotype. Int J Cancer 54:1010–1016
14. Mercier I et al (2008) Human breast cancer-associated fibroblasts (CAFs) show caveolin-1 downregulation and RB tumor suppressor functional inactivation: Implications for the response to hormonal therapy. Cancer Biol Ther 7:1212–1225
15. Olumi AF et al (1999) Carcinoma-associated fibroblasts direct tumor progression of initiated human prostatic epithelium. Cancer Res 59:5002–5011
16. Hwang RF et al (2008) Cancer-associated stromal fibroblasts promote pancreatic tumor progression. Cancer Res 68:918–926
17. Barcellos-Hoff MH, Ravani SA (2000) Irradiated mammary gland stroma promotes the expression of tumorigenic potential by unirradiated epithelial cells. Cancer Res 60:1254–1260
18. Orimo A, Weinberg RA (2007) Heterogeneity of stromal fibroblasts in tumors. Cancer Biol Ther 6:618–619
19. Sugimoto H, Mundel TM, Kieran MW, Kalluri R (2006) Identification of fibroblast heterogeneity in the tumor microenvironment. Cancer Biol Ther 5:1640–1646
20. Ronnov-Jessen L, Petersen OW, Bissell MJ (1996) Cellular changes involved in conversion of normal to malignant breast: importance of the stromal reaction. Physiol Rev 76:69–125
21. Serini G, Gabbiani G (1999) Mechanisms of myofibroblast activity and phenotypic modulation. Exp Cell Res 250:273–283
22. Roberts AB et al (1986) Transforming growth factor type beta: rapid induction of fibrosis and angiogenesis in vivo and stimulation of collagen formation in vitro. Proc Natl Acad Sci USA 83:4167–4171
23. Direkze NC et al (2004) Bone marrow contribution to tumor-associated myofibroblasts and fibroblasts. Cancer Res 64:8492–8495

24. Ishii G et al (2003) Bone-marrow-derived myofibroblasts contribute to the cancer-induced stromal reaction. Biochem Biophys Res Commun 309:232–240
25. Mishra PJ et al (2008) Carcinoma-associated fibroblast-like differentiation of human mesenchymal stem cells. Cancer Res 68:4331–4339
26. Iwano M et al (2002) Evidence that fibroblasts derive from epithelium during tissue fibrosis. J Clin Invest 110:341–350
27. Zeisberg EM, Potenta S, Xie L, Zeisberg M, Kalluri R (2007) Discovery of endothelial to mesenchymal transition as a source for carcinoma-associated fibroblasts. Cancer Res 67: 10123–10128
28. Folkman J (1995) Angiogenesis in cancer, vascular, rheumatoid and other disease. Nat Med 1:27–31
29. Sun J et al (2004) Blocking angiogenesis and tumorigenesis with GFA-116, a synthetic molecule that inhibits binding of vascular endothelial growth factor to its receptor. Cancer Res 64:3586–3592
30. Orimo A et al (2005) Stromal fibroblasts present in invasive human breast carcinomas promote tumor growth and angiogenesis through elevated SDF-1/CXCL12 secretion. Cell 121: 335–348
31. Guo X, Oshima H, Kitmura T, Taketo MM, Oshima M (2008) Stromal fibroblasts activated by tumor cells promote angiogenesis in mouse gastric cancer. J Biol Chem 283:19864–19871
32. Razani B, Lisanti MP (2001) Caveolin-deficient mice: insights into caveolar function and human disease. J Clin Invest 108:1553–1561
33. Mercier I et al (2009) Clinical and translational implications of the caveolin gene family: lessons from mouse models and human genetic disorders. Lab Invest 89(6):614–623
34. Koleske AJ, Baltimore D, Lisanti MP (1995) Reduction of caveolin and caveolae in oncogenically transformed cells. Proc Natl Acad Sci USA 92:1381–1385
35. Galbiati F et al (2001) Caveolin-1 expression negatively regulates cell cycle progression by inducing G(0)/G(1) arrest via a p53/p21(WAF1/Cip1)-dependent mechanism. Mol Biol Cell 12:2229–2244
36. Torres VA et al (2006) Caveolin-1 controls cell proliferation and cell death by suppressing expression of the inhibitor of apoptosis protein survivin. J Cell Sci 119:1812–1823
37. Weinberg RA (1995) The retinoblastoma protein and cell cycle control. Cell 81:323–330
38. Gratton JP et al (2003) Selective inhibition of tumor microvascular permeability by cavtratin blocks tumor progression in mice. Cancer Cell 4:31–39
39. Jasmin JF, Mercier I, Dupuis J, Tanowitz HB, Lisanti MP (2006) Short-term administration of a cell-permeable caveolin-1 peptide prevents the development of monocrotaline-induced pulmonary hypertension and right ventricular hypertrophy. Circulation 114:912–920
40. Ross JS (2009) Multigene classifiers, prognostic factors, and predictors of breast cancer clinical outcome. Adv Anat Pathol 16:204–215
41. Witkiewicz AK et al (2009) An absence of stromal caveolin-1 expression predicts early tumor recurrence and poor clinical outcome in human breast cancers. Am J Pathol 174:2023 2034
42. Sloan EK et al (2009) Stromal cell expression of caveolin-1 predicts outcome in breast cancer. Am J Pathol 174:2035–2043
43. Patani N, Cutuli B, Mokbel K (2008) Current management of DCIS: a review. Breast Cancer Res Treat 111:1–10
44. Witkiewicz AK et al (2009) Stromal caveolin-1 levels predict early DCIS progression to invasive breast cancer. Cancer Biol Ther 8:1071–1079
45. Di Vizio D et al (2009) An absence of stromal caveolin-1 is associated with advanced prostate cancer, metastatic disease and epithelial Akt activation. Cell Cycle 8:2420–2424
46. McCall P, Gemmell LK, Mukherjee R, Bartlett JM, Edwards J (2008) Phosphorylation of the androgen receptor is associated with reduced survival in hormone-refractory prostate cancer patients. Br J Cancer 98:1094–1101
47. Mike S et al (2006) Chemotherapy for hormone-refractory prostate cancer. Cochrane Database Syst Rev (4):CD005247

48. Williams TM et al (2006) Stromal and epithelial caveolin-1 both confer a protective effect against mammary hyperplasia and tumorigenesis: caveolin-1 antagonizes cyclin D1 function in mammary epithelial cells. Am J Pathol 169(5):1784–1801
49. Mercier I et al (2009) Genetic ablation of caveolin-1 drives estrogen-hypersensitivity and the development of DCIS-like mammary lesions. Am J Pathol 174:1172–1190
50. Sotgia F et al (2009) Caveolin-1−/− null mammary stromal fibroblasts share characteristics with human breast cancer-associated fibroblasts. Am J Pathol 174:746–761

Index

A

Adenomatous polyposis coli (APC), 19
Angiogenesis, 75–76. *See also* Tumor
    angiogenesis

B

Brain tumors
    glial cells and brain vessels, 53
    glioma vasculature, 59
    molecular interface, 59–60
    neoplastic cells
        astrocytic tumors, 55
        breast carcinomas, 56
        EGFR sequestration, 55
        human glioblastoma cell lines, 54
        immunofluorescence analyses, 54
        mesenchymal phenotype, 57
        oligodendroglial tumors, 57–59
Breast cancer
    apoptosis process, 95–96
    cellular adhesion, 92
    D7S522 locus, 91
    mammary tumorigenesis, 92–94
    metastasis formation, 95
    tumor metabolism, 96–98

C

Cancer-associated stromal fibroblasts
    caveolin–1
        cancer stroma, 109–110
        DCIS lesions, 114
        HRPC status, 114
        immunofluorescence analysis, 116
        myofibroblast-like morphology, 115
        paracrine mechanisms, 116

        stromal-targeted therapies,
          110–112
        tamoxifen-resistance, 112
        tissue microarrays, 112
    source and origin, 108
    tumor angiogenesis, 109
    tumor growth, 106–108
    wound healing, 105
Carcinoembryonic antigen-related cell
    adhesion molecule 6
    (CEACAM6), 45
Castrate-resistant PCa (CRPC), 2, 6
β-catenin
    actin cytoskeleton, 23
    APC, 19
    Axin, 20
    ectopic expression, 22
    immunoprecipitation, 22
    oncogenes, 19
    plasma membrane, 23
Caveolin–1 (Cav–1)
    brain tumors
        astrocytic tumors, 55
        breast carcinomas, 56
        EGFR sequestration, 55
        glial cells and brain vessels, 53
        glioma vasculature, 59
        human glioblastoma cell lines, 54
        immunofluorescence analyses, 54
        mesenchymal phenotype, 57
        molecular interface, 59–60
        oligodendroglial tumors, 57–59
    breast cancer
        apoptosis process, 95–96
        cyclin D1 gene, 92
        D7S522 locus, 91
        estrogens, 93

I. Mercier et al. (eds.), *Caveolins in Cancer Pathogenesis, Prevention and Therapy,*
Current Cancer Research, DOI 10.1007/978-1-4614-1001-0,
© Springer Science+Business Media, LLC 2012

Caveolin–1 (Cav–1) (*cont.*)
    mammary epithelial cell hyperplasia, 92
    metastasis formation, 95
    prolactin, 94
    tumor metabolism, 96–98
  cancer stroma
    DCIS lesions, 114
    HRPC status, 114
    immunofluorescence analysis, 116
    myofibroblast-like morphology, 115
    paracrine mechanisms, 116
    stromal-targeted therapies, 110–112
    tamoxifen-resistance, 112
    tissue microarrays, 112
  colon cancer
    β-catenin-Tcf/Lef target gene, 25
    canonical Wnt signaling, 26
    COX–2, 25, 26
    epigenetic mechanisms, 27
    human colorectal carcinoma cell
      lines, 30
    intestinal tissues, 29
    methotrexate, 31
    PGE_2, 26
    plasma membrane, 24
    survivin expression, 24
    tissue analysis, 28
    transcriptional regulation, 27
    tumorigenesis, 32, 33
  pancreatic ductal adenocarcinoma
    anchorage-independent cell survival, 45
    CEACAM6 crosslinking, 45
    ectopic expression, 44
    FASN, 47
    pathogenesis, 45–47
    reverse Warburg effect, 44
    targeted therapy, 49
    tumorigenesis, 49
  prostate cancer
    local tumor microenvironment, 8–9
    metastatic tumor microenvironment,
      9–10
    oncogenic activities, 6–7
    overexpression, 4–6
    prostatic epithelial cells, 4
    secretion of, 7–8
    stromal cells, 3
    tumor progression, 4
    tumor suppressor gene, 3
  skin cancer
    cancer dissemination, 71
    exosomes, 66, 71
    gastric carcinoma, 67
    human melanoma cells, 66

    lymph node metastases, 68
    membrane fusion mechanism, 71
    metastatic-secreted vesicles, 70
    paracrine diffusion, 72
    phosphorylation status, 69
    sphingolipids, 72
    tumor cells, 69
Colon cancer
  canonical Wnt signaling
    actin cytoskeleton, 23
    APC, 19
    Axin, 20
    β-catenin, 20
    ectopic expression, 22
    immunoprecipitation, 22
    oncogenes, 19
    plasma membrane, 23
  caveolin–1
    human colon cancer cell lines,
      28–31
    tissue analysis, 28
    tumor suppressor, 23–27
  cell migration, 18
  multidrug resistance, 18
Colorectal cancer. *See* Wnt signaling
Cyclooxygenase–2 (COX–2), 25

D
Ductal carcinomas in situ (DCIS), 114

E
Endothelial cell (EC), 75

F
Fatty acid synthase (FASN), 47
Fibroblast growth factor (FGF), 76

G
Ganglioside sphingo lipid (GSL), 67
Genitourinary (GU) tract, 1

H
Hormone refractory prostate cancer
    (HRPC), 114
Human umbilical vein EC (HUVEC), 82

L
Lewis lung carcinoma (LLC), 84

M
Melanoma. *See* Skin cancer
Microvascular density (MVD), 82

P
Pancreatic ductal adenocarcinoma (PDA)
 caveolin–1
  anchorage-independent cell
   survival, 45
  biomarker, 47–49
  CEACAM6 crosslinking, 45
  ectopic expression, 44
  pathogenesis, 45–47
  reverse Warburg effect, 44
  targeted therapy, 49
 genetic mutations, 43
 overexpressed genes, 44
 surgical resection, 43
Proliferating cell nuclear antigen (PCNA), 112
Prostaglandin E_2 (PGE$_2$), 26
Prostate cancer (PCa)
 androgen deprivation, 1
 caveolin–1
  local tumor microenvironment, 8–9
  metastatic tumor microenvironment,
   9–10
  oncogenic activities, 6–7
  overexpression, 4–6
  prostatic epithelial cells, 4
  secretion of, 7–8
  stromal cells, 3
  tumor progression, 4
  tumor suppressor gene, 3
 GU tract, 1

R
Radical prostatectomy, 4

S
Skin cancer
 anchorage dependent cell growth, 66
 caveolin–1
  cancer dissemination, 71
  exosomes, 66, 71
  gastric carcinoma, 67
  human melanoma cells, 66

lymph node metastases, 68
  membrane fusion mechanism, 71
  metastatic-secreted vesicles, 70
  paracrine diffusion, 72
  phosphorylation status, 69
  sphingolipids, 72
  tumor cells, 69
 scaffolding domain, 65
 tumor suppressor, 65
Suppressor of cytokine signaling–1
 (SOCS–1), 94

T
Tumor angiogenesis
 angiogenic switch
  EC proliferation, 75
  pro-and antiangiogenic factors, 76
 caveolin–1
  B16-F1 melanoma cells, 77
  capillary tube formation, 82
  clinical studies, 83, 86
  EC proliferation, 87
  EC signaling, 77
  fibrinogen, 84
  hepatic cell carcinoma, 83
  LLC cells, 84
  LNCaP cells, 79
  matrigel, 87
  MVD, 82
  negative role, in vitro assays, 85–86
  positive role, in vitro assays, 79–82
  pro-and antiangiogenic factors, 86–87

V
Vascular endothelial growth factor (VEGF), 76

W
Wnt signaling
 actin cytoskeleton, 23
 APC, 19
 axin, 20
 β-catenin, 20
 ectopic expression, 22
 immunoprecipitation, 22
 oncogenes, 19
 plasma membrane, 23